THE LOVING CAREGIVER

THE LOVING CAREGIVER

Two People Face Back-To-Back Crises Hand In Hand

BY ALICE AND AMBROSE DUDLEY

CHAPEL HILL
PRESS, INC.

Front cover photo © Alice H. Dudley.
Back cover photo taken when Alice and Ambrose
were vacationing in the Canadian Rockies.

Rancho Los Amigos Levels of Cognitive Function reprinted with the permission of Rancho
Los Amigos.
Excerpt from sermon by the Rev. Harold M. Robinson reprinted with the permission of
Harold M. Robinson, Jr.
"A New Way of Struggling" by Dr. Susan W. N. Ruach used with the permission of the author.
God Calling daily devotionals reprinted with the permission of Barbour Publishing, Inc.

ISBN-10: 1-59715-026-6
ISBN-13: 978-1-59715-026-2
Library of Congress Catalog Number 2006930935

First Printing

To
Barbara & George
Two long-Time loving
Caregivers. *[signature]* & Alice

It takes a circle of care to fight
a major disease or injury

CONTENTS

MEET THE CAREGIVERS

This book is about two people and how they victoriously handled back-to-back crises with love, understanding, and care. And how they were comforted and sustained by a circle of care.

It is left to others to tell about the mechanics of fighting an aggressive form of cancer and the medical details of dealing with a severe brain injury. This book touches briefly on details of the illness and injury and the medical expertise used to treat them only to help the reader understand what happened.

We are Alice and Ambrose. Our goal is to tell the story of the caregiver from the inside out—from the frontlines—in the hope that our experiences will be helpful to others who, God forbid, find themselves in similar situations.

We each will tell different parts of the story, and we will try to make it clear who is speaking. Some parts will be told jointly, as is this prologue, to *The Loving Caregiver*. We see the word *caregiver* as a representation of how we cared for each other and how God cared for both of us through others.

Alice was the caregiver for Ambrose after he was diagnosed in February 1997 with multiple myeloma, a cancer that causes plasma cells in the bone marrow to replicate wildly. Ambrose underwent a stem cell transplant

(SCT), sometimes called a bone marrow transplant (BMT), in September/ October of 1997.

Ambrose was the caregiver for Alice after she suffered a severe brain injury in a traffic accident in April 1999. She was in a coma for nearly three weeks and underwent daily rehabilitative therapy for more than a year.

From the first word of Ambrose's illness and Alice's accident the circle of care began to form around us. We felt the love of family, friends, and associates from far and wide. That circle of care included concern not only for patient, but for the caregiver.

We felt very fortunate to have such a caring community. The circle of care included prayer, visitations, meals, and help with the daily routine of running a household.

The kindness shown by doctors, family, friends, and associates was crucial to the healing process. Ambrose was deeply touched when a meeting of his peers in New York City included a prayer service for him. The bar in the hospitality suite became an altar, and prayers of love were lifted up for his healing.

That is what this book is about: People caring for people and how this care empowers the patient and the caregiver as they fight the battle for life.

INTRODUCTION

By Jane Kincheloe McDonald

The time had come at our daughter's wedding rehearsal dinner party for a toast from the bride's family. The preceding roasts had delighted the beaming couple, and they waited expectantly for the closing maternal admonition and blessing.

To their surprise, I turned to another couple, each with a benevolent posture and knowing smile. I directed the room's attention toward them.

"This is the way a marriage looks when you keep the vows you will make tomorrow," I said to the prospective bride and groom. "You do not know what your future holds, but you will pledge to love and cherish for better or for worse, in sickness and in health. Here is a couple that daily lives out their promise to God and each other."

I introduced Alice and Ambrose and briefly shared their challenging experiences. There was a long applause.

When I first met Ambrose, I was amused by this pipe-chomping, intense young man who acted like life's ticker tape was moving too slowly. In contrast, his Kentucky drawl made every conversation seem folksy and most interesting. He was an early-rising, "two-cup regular" type of person who routinely began each day with "quiet time" with the Lord. He was the consummate provider for his family. He would build fires on cold New England days for their comfort and pleasure and in due season proudly present to them abundant harvests from his garden. O yes, he was also the bureau chief of the Associated Press in Connecticut.

Alice immediately impressed me as the world's best mother, friend, and cook. I've never changed my mind. Beneath the everyday chatter, usually over a cup of tea at four o'clock via telephone, were the "givens" of our mirrored lives. Our mutual commitment to the Lord made us sisters.

In summary, I could say that Alice and Ambrose enjoyed very busy lives but lived each day against the backdrop of eternity. It was good to have such friends.

Like salmon, completing life's cycle, Alice and Ambrose returned to the South. We headed for the Midwest. New lives and new friends enveloped us, but the memories of our times together lay like tissue-wrapped treasures in the trunks of our hearts. Anytime we wished, we could dust off the memory and enjoy it again. We lived our lives believing that the circle of life would bring us back together.

We did not expect the phone call in 1997. Ambrose had been diagnosed with multiple myeloma. The words ran together—hopeful, procedures, transplants, isolation, very serious. Ambrose had prayed for us on several critical occasions, and now we'd pray for him and summon others to do the same. He experienced it all, and then came the news—clean diagnosis. We were amazed by his courage and by our God!

The truck came from nowhere in April 1999. Alice was on her way to a required school workshop. Alice, as we knew her, was changed. The helper now needed the help.

She remained unconscious for weeks—the prayer warriors assumed their positions. "Thy will be done,—Amen." Her eyes eventually opened, and so did life's opportunities.

As I studied my two friends slowly dancing and holding each other at our daughter's wedding, I marveled. They didn't just survive. They seemed to thrive. What's their secret? Here is their story with a valuable look at life's learned lessons.

(Jane lives in Mariemont, Ohio)

ONE

AMBROSE: Alice had tears in her eyes when we turned from the altar of the little Methodist church in Yadkinville, North Carolina "I cried, too," I whispered to her as we walked out into a chilly November afternoon in 1964 to begin to construct something new.

Our tears were tears of joy, although mine could have been because my pants were too short and too tight.

The joy came from the vows we had just spoken to each other from memory. We promised ourselves to each other in sickness and in health. Little did we know what that would mean for the two of us.

Before us in the next forty-two years were a battle with cancer and recovery from a closed head injury within a twenty-six-month period. How we handled those twin life-threatening events would test our faith and our marriage vows.

Although we had no way of knowing exactly what was ahead of us, major struggles undoubtedly were on the mind of the minister who counseled us before marriage. The minister was Alice's uncle, Dr. Robert G. Tuttle.

He told us that when we said the vows we would be creating something brand new: a marriage. He added that our marriage would survive if we remembered that there were three parties in the covenant: Alice, Ambrose, and God.

Dr. Tuttle said we should always keep God in the center of our marriage. If we did that, he predicted we would have a happy and fulfilling marriage and we would be able to deal with the problems and struggles life would send our way. He also encouraged us to pray and always say, "I love you" before going about each day's tasks.

The little town of Yadkinville in the western Piedmont of North Carolina was Alice's home. She grew up there before leaving for college at High Point University and then working as a director of Christian education in the big city of Charlotte.

Her dad, Fred Colby Hobson, was the superintendent of schools in Yadkin County for more than thirty years. Her mother, Miriam Tuttle Hobson, worked in the home and was a tower of strength in the Methodist church. Miriam's father was a Methodist minister, as was her brother, Robert. Bob and Miriam had a sibling, Emily, who was a college English teacher.

I grew up in Frankfort, Kentucky, where my father, Ambrose, was in real estate and insurance. He served terms on the city council and was deputy mayor at one point. He was widely known for a radio show he and the local Sears manager did each year to raise money for the March of Dimes.

Dad and Mom both took major roles in the Frankfort Methodist Church.

My mother, Lucretia, was a schoolteacher. Her father was a Methodist minister in Western Kentucky.

After high school, I attended the University of Kentucky. I was more interested in watching the basketball team win games (including a NCAA championship in 1958) than studying. After a couple of disastrous semesters, I was asked to stay out of school for a semester.

During that time I found work in various places including at the local newspaper, the *State Journal*, soon moving from the advertising department selling ads for a special edition to news editor in the editorial department.

I returned to college part-time at night but soon realized the science requirements were beyond my abilities to comprehend. I had a decision to make: either stay in school and try to learn the parts of the frog or begin a career in journalism. I chose the latter.

I was offered a temporary job helping to cover the North Carolina General Assembly for The Associated Press. The pay was more than twice the $50 a week I was making at the *State Journal*, and the position could lead to a career.

I withdrew from the University of Kentucky and promised my mother I could complete my degree someday in the future. I prepared to leave for North Carolina the third week in January.

There was one more bit of business I needed to tend to in Frankfort. My friend for sixteen years, a collie-shepherd named Mr. Chips, had cancer and was not expected to live long. We decided that he should be put out of his misery. I dug a grave with tears rolling down my cheeks. The vet came to our house, administered a drug, and carried Mr. Chips to his final resting-place.

The next week I left for North Carolina. After four months of covering the legislature in Raleigh, the AP offered me another temporary job in Charlotte.

It was there in Dilworth Methodist Church that I met Alice. She was director of children's work at Dilworth and a member of the choir, which sang from a raised loft behind the pulpit. The pastor, the Reverend Harold M. Robinson, was a big man with a booming voice.

Alice had a habit of falling asleep during his sermons. I had to meet this person who could sleep through one of Pastor Robinson's robust sermons. We started dating a few months after we met. We felt we were right for each other. We decided to get married in November after I was transferred to a regular AP job in Raleigh.

Alice went home to Yadkinville to plan the wedding instead of taking a new job with Mouzon Methodist Church in Charlotte.

Following a honeymoon in Williamsburg, Virginia, we moved to Raleigh, where I worked for the AP and Alice was director of Christian education at Hayes Barton Methodist Church. We moved back to Charlotte eighteen months later, and Alice found that Mouzon Methodist Church again needed a director of Christian education.

It was in Charlotte that our marriage faced its first real test. We wanted to have a baby but were not successful. It was my problem, the doctors said. We tried and we tried. The pressure was building because having a child was an enormous issue in Alice's way of thinking.

I wanted children, too, but I wasn't driven as Alice was. Anyway, we prayed and prayed. It took a few years before Alice realized success was on the way. Our marriage had cleared a major hurdle.

We wanted to have natural childbirth with the daddy in the delivery room. After finding a doctor who would agree to that arrangement, we learned there was only one hospital in Charlotte that would hear of such a thing.

We took childbirth education classes, learning to pant and blow and work as a team. We headed for Mercy Hospital at 8 a.m. April 11, 1969. It was a hard day of work for Alice and me.

We almost gave up around 6 p.m. because Alice was so tired, but when the nurse said Alice had finally dilated significantly, we got a new burst of energy. The baby, Gregory, was born at 7:14 p.m. and weighed 7 pounds, 14 ounces. He was always a perfectionist.

Two months later, the AP offered me a transfer to Providence, Rhode Island, as correspondent. I was so anxious to move up the ladder that I accepted immediately. I got off the telephone and asked Alice, "Where is Providence?"

We headed for Rhode Island. We learned the New England ways and found many good friends. In two years, we wanted to have another child. We knew it might take a while for Alice to get pregnant based on the experience with Greg.

It didn't. Christopher was soon on the way. So was the moving van. The AP transferred us to Hartford in central Connecticut for a news editor position.

The doctors and hospitals in Connecticut opened their arms to natural childbirth and the father being in the delivery room. Since Greg had been so slow in being born, Alice felt there was no need to hurry when contractions began in earnest.

I disagreed, and we headed for St. Francis Hospital. Alice's water broke when she got to the hospital. The doctor let out an expletive, and Alice was rushed to the delivery room. Things happened fast. The nurse tossed me a gown and shoes and said, "Follow me, quickly!"

We knew that Christopher had not settled headfirst into the birth canal. The doctors could not tell his position. So we had broken water and a baby in an unknown position.

The umbilical cord was the first part that was visible. The doctor, who declared "Let's go; I am going to deliver the baby," kept the cord in one hand and looked for a part of the baby with the other.

He found a foot first. Christopher was a footling breech with a prolapsed cord. The doctor pulled him out while Alice dug her fingers into my arms.

Chris was so tired from the delivery that he was limp in the doctor's hand. I thought that he was dead. My heart sank. The doctor said to wait a minute, that he was okay. And he was.

I was so nervous that I backed into a car in a downtown parking lot. It was only the second accident I'd ever had that was my fault.

I became chief of bureau for the Connecticut AP, a post I held for eight years. Alice was a stay-at-home mom and then a part-time preschool teacher. We accepted a transfer back to Raleigh in 1980. We loved our years in New England, but I had shoveled enough snow. We left some great friends in New England and went home.

It was great to be home again. I grew up in Kentucky but adopted North Carolina as my second home. I love the state and really appreciate the fact Raleigh is three and a half hours from the coast at Pine Knoll Shores where Alice's sister, Jane, and her husband, Bill, live and from the mountains of Ashe County where our family owns a cottage overlooking the New River.

Once the boys got older, Alice wanted to work outside the home and took a job as a teacher's assistant. She enjoyed the people she worked with and the pupils but felt she had more to offer. She decided that being an elementary school guidance counselor would be the best use of her talents.

She started taking a course or two at North Carolina State University in Raleigh. It reminded me that I still had not completed college and needed to do so. But for now the whole focus was on getting Alice into graduate school.

She succeeded after impressing the people at NCSU by doing well in the night courses she took. She became a full-time graduate student just as Greg was finishing his third year at High Point University and Chris about to enroll there as a freshman.

We had three family members in college at the same time. We didn't need a fourth. I had taken a course at Wake Technical Community College in human resources. I saw this as a test to see if the old brain could retain enough to get by. I knew it was not the time to go back to school in earnest.

The loss of one salary and having three people in college at once was a real struggle financially. Alice's sister, Jane, helped to pay for Alice's education, and we just buckled down.

It was worth it. Alice graduated with a master's in education in May 1991. She had done her internship in the Wake County public schools and thought that would be a good place to find a job.

Her efforts were met with the unbelievable excuses of "We wanted a younger person," "We want someone who lives close to the school," "We need a man for this position," "We need a black to balance the staff," and on and on.

Finally, Mike Ward, superintendent of schools in Granville County and later state superintendent of public instruction, hired Alice to fill in for a counselor on sick leave at Butner-Stem Elementary in Butner, site of a federal correctional institute and some of the state's mental health hospitals.

A year later she was given the job as a regular position. Alice loved working with the children. The schools use their counselors for many non-counseling jobs such as end-of-grade test administrator, testing coordinator, and meeting attender.

Alice was to represent Butner-Stem at a state-mandated workshop on how to care for handicapped children when disaster struck.

AMBROSE RETURNS TO SCHOOL

With Alice out of college, I had decided it was time for me to return to the classroom. I had taken courses in the noncredit Lay Academy at Duke Divinity School in nearby Durham. I had gotten to know one of the professors, Dr. James M. (Mickey) Efird. We discussed my possibly going into the ministry late in life, and he suggested I resume my schooling at Meredith College in Raleigh where he had a professor friend.

The friend said that wouldn't work because Meredith was an all-women's college, something we had forgotten. The friend suggested a program in Raleigh run by North Carolina Wesleyan College (NCWC) in Rocky Mount.

I enrolled in the adult education program in the spring of 1992 and was frightened that the problems I had in my early college career would reappear and that I would not have the mental capacity to do the work and remember details long enough to successfully finish a test.

I took a course in communication skills first, figuring that with my writing and speaking background I might get through this one. I was a nervous wreck for the first test. The instructor, a doctoral student at NCSU, was a wonderful instructor. I enjoyed the course, flourished, and made an A.

I took one or two classes a semester and was in no hurry to finish school. Many of my courses from the University of Kentucky did not transfer to NCWC. I received credit for 81 hours and needed 49 to graduate. That is a steep hill for a 52-year-old person to face.

There were some really wonderful instructors from the community in the program. It was great to have people who did this stuff for a living teaching courses on economics, statistics, business law, business finance, and human resources. They could relate everyday experiences to explain material in the textbooks.

I was deep in the NCWC program, taking a course in art appreciation, when I was diagnosed with cancer.

Life took a sudden turn for us.

Alice and I learned plenty in rearing two boys, and we felt our formal education in later life was most valuable. We considered ourselves much richer for having gone back to school.

However, nothing could have prepared us for what lay ahead. You only learn as you live through it.

TWO

And who knows whether you have not come to
the Kingdom for such a time as this.
Esther 4:14 (RSV)

AMBROSE: Twin disasters struck within twenty-six months. I was diagnosed with cancer in February 1997, and Alice suffered a severe brain injury in an automobile accident in April 1999.

"For better, for worse ... in sickness and health," our marital vows said. We were now going to get to test the strength of those vows.

And we were going to learn a new skill: caring for a person in a life-threatening situation. This task was thrust upon us. We didn't apply for it. The job came without training and without warning.

We learned that caregivers, like Queen Esther, find themselves suddenly faced with an opportunity to serve in a way they never planned. Their new role in life often pushes their abilities and patience to the limit. They must learn a new trade on the job.

We also had another job, that of patient. We at least had had some experience in this role, but we had none as the caregiver for a person in a life-threatening situation.

We learned quickly that the job of caregiver is key for the healing process and for the patient's general well-being. We also realized what Dr. Tuttle had meant when he said to keep God in the center of our marriage. God is the most loving caregiver.

Alice cared for me after I was diagnosed with multiple myeloma (MM), a cancer that causes plasma cells in the bone marrow to replicate wildly.

I underwent a peripheral stem cell transplant in September/October of 1997 at UNC Hospitals in Chapel Hill, NC. (The procedure is sometimes called a bone marrow transplant, which is really something else. We will refer to it as a transplant or stem cell transplant [SCT].

Twenty-six months later it was my turn. I cared for Alice after she suffered a brain injury in a traffic accident. She was in a coma for nearly three weeks and underwent daily rehabilitative therapy for more than a year.

Friends were shocked, of course; as were we.

"How much can one couple be asked to bear?" was a common question among friends, relatives, and associates as word of Alice's accident spread.

Eight years later, we are continuing to support and care for each other.

Alice struggles to find new ways to deal with the deficits caused by her brain injury, and I live with debilitating fatigue and under a cloud of uncertainty. The word *cure* is not used by my doctors in connection with MM.

I am convinced that we have made it this far because of the vows we made in 1964 to be there for each other. When trouble came, we never wanted to do anything else but care for each other — even though it was very difficult and heart-breaking at times.

We found that the caregiver shoulders the heaviest load. The patient is busy with consequences of the illness/injury and the medical treatment. That occupies his or her time and thoughts.

As the caregiver, we had to simply watch as our loved one struggled to regain a quality and a wholeness of life. There is a helpless feeling when the patient is really struggling and there is little more the caregiver or the doctors can do while waiting for the body and the brain to heal.

We were exhausted at times. The caregiver is always on call and must stand ready to respond at a moment's notice regardless of how tired he or she feels. We learned to live with inconveniences and disruptions. We also learned to stand back at times and let others carry the load.

Since the role of caregiver can be almost mind-bending, we wanted to make provisions for taking care of ourselves.

We quickly realized that the wise caregiver includes as part of the recovery plan a schedule to get away from the immediate situation of caring for the patient and to care for his- or herself. We used a telephone tree to spread the latest word on the patient's condition, thus conserving our energy.

I scheduled trips to the beach and to the mountains at intervals during Alice's early recovery. Later, when Alice could travel, we planned breaks in her therapy for vacations. Her primary rehabilitation doctor, Dr. Patrick O'Brien, encouraged this. At certain periods he declared it was time for a break.

Alice found relief from the daily grind of caring for me by retreating to the homes of her brother, Fred, or our son, Chris, both of whom lived near UNC Hospitals at the time. I encouraged her to do so. She also frequently went to lunch or dinner with friends.

That was one of the advantages of having an inpatient SCT. Alice could get time away for rest and renewal because nurses cared for me.

More and more, transplants are being done on an outpatient basis. The patient and the caregiver spend the night and much of the day at a nearby apartment and return to the hospital only for treatment. This allows little or no time for the caregiver to sleep or relax.

We were fortunate to have a number of friends who helped take care of us. We felt the love of family, friends, and associates from near and far.

Our caring community prayed for us, visited us, provided food, and helped in the daily chores of running a household. We didn't have the time or the energy to do many things that were once routine. We were busy trying to figure out how to deal with the medical crisis before us.

With the help of friends who had fought major medical battles themselves, I developed a mantra for dealing with an illness or a major medical crisis. It served Alice and me well during both treatments. It had these elements:

> *Trust* your doctor to know what to do and how to handle the situation. Don't try to play doctor.
> *Trust* the treatment plan you and your doctor work out.
> *Trust* your body to work to heal itself, if you don't hinder it with negative thoughts.
> *Trust* your God to be with you throughout, if you will allow Him to be.

We learned to weed out anything that can slow, stop, or hinder treatment and recovery. A primary hindrance to recovery is the lack of a positive attitude about life.

Shortly after I began cancer treatment, I received from a newspaper colleague a book titled *You Can't Afford the Luxury of a Negative Thought* by John-Roger and Peter McWilliams (Prelude Press, 1991). It explained the power of positive thought and the ruinous effects of negative thought.

Dr. Don Gabriel of UNC Hospitals said my positive attitude during the cancer treatment was equal to another round of chemo in helping my healing.

A major element in Alice's recovery was her positive attitude and determination to win the battle.

The hundreds of cards, letters, and other expressions of love we received were uplifting to us. Knowing that our friends were thinking of us strengthened our resolve to win.

The random acts of kindness shown by doctors, family, friends, and associates were crucial to the healing process.

We learned that caring people empower the patient and the caregiver as they fight the battle for life. We will always be deeply indebted to those who gave so much that we might concentrate our efforts on getting well.

The struggle was hourly in both of our cases. We feel that going through the twin battles made us stronger individuals, a stronger couple, and more sensitive people to those who are suffering.

THREE

ALICE: It started with a simple bump against the sharp edge of a wooden bookshelf in his office as Ambrose was rushing to the AP newsroom to check on a breaking story.

There was no reason to be concerned. If he had cracked a rib, what would doctors do? Let it heal since wrapping it could lead to pneumonia. At least that is what he thought on that March day in 1996.

The rib still hurt in July, and Ambrose made an appointment with his doctor. He was examined by a physician's assistant since his doctor was on vacation. She ordered an x-ray. The report: Ambrose had re-injured his rib.

Hurricane Fran hit the Raleigh area in September, and Ambrose joined the men in our neighborhood in trying to clean up the mess. He helped cut trees, carry limbs and logs, and tried to be of assistance where he could. He was tired but thought nothing of it.

He did comment to his administrative assistant weeks later that he wished someone would tell him why he was so tired all the time. His annual physical exam showed he was anemic. His red blood count was low. Some tests were ordered and reordered in a few months.

When diagnosis could not be made, Ambrose was referred to a

hematologist/oncologist, Dr. Virgil Rose. He examined Ambrose in mid-February 1997, performed a bone marrow biopsy, and ordered x-rays of every bone in his body.

Two days later Dr. Rose called with the results: *cancer*. The type: multiple myeloma, IgA, stage 3. The disease had taken over Ambrose's body.

We went to the Internet to find out what we were dealing with. A 1996 publication for doctors by the International Myeloma Foundation (IMF) said:

> Multiple Myeloma (MM) is a malignancy of plasma cells, occurring usually in the bone marrow, but sometimes in other body sites. The clinical picture of multiple Myeloma is varied and has a number of characteristic features including bone destruction with bone pain, elevated levels of paraprotein in serum and Bence Jones proteins in urine, anemia, elevated serum calcium and impaired renal function."(myeloma.org)

The disease is life-threatening. There is no known cure.

Dr. Rose said he would order a chemotherapy drug for Ambrose as a starter and we should make an appointment for a follow-up visit. Ambrose began the chemo treatment immediately, envisioning the pills going through his body gobbling up the cancer cells.

We were stunned, of course. Life had taken a sudden change for us. We needed to consider how to handle this crisis of crises in our marriage.

We notified the family and close friends and put Ambrose on our church's prayer list. We turned to God in prayer. We asked guidance in how to deal with the situation. We also expressed thanksgiving for life itself and God's presence in the midst of crises.

Ambrose decided to keep an appointment in the northeastern part of the state the day after we got *the news*. It was a three-and-a-half-hour drive each way. He needed the time alone in the car to think and sort things out. It was a wise move. He came back from the trip more focused and determined to fight.

He called the AP's home office in New York City to tell them of the diagnosis and that he would have to be on sick leave for a while. His bosses were very supportive.

I told people at the school where I was a guidance counselor. Their love encompassed me. Teachers and administrators at Butner-Stem Elementary offered to "give" me their sick days so I could be away longer without losing pay.

We didn't know what was ahead of us, but we knew we wouldn't face it alone. We knew we were loved. The old and worn phrase that we had heard so much kept popping up in our minds: *We don't know what the future holds, but we know* Who *holds the future.*

It is interesting how things you have heard all your life come back to you at the very moment you need them. It is like there is an invisible hand guiding you.

Ambrose was one of 39,500 people in North Carolina and 1.4 million in the United States diagnosed with cancer that year. Of those, 13,800 were diagnosed with MM.

The statistics on survival were not encouraging. Without treatment, Ambrose could expect to live about seven months. With conventional chemo, he was given from nine to sixty months, depending on the number of cancer cells in his body. He had a bunch of them.

Ambrose was diagnosed to be in stage 3 (the worst stage) of MM. The biopsy showed that 90 percent of his bone marrow contained sheets of plasma cells gone amok. Usually, plasma cells make up only 3–5 percent of the bone marrow.

Ambrose was a sick little boy at age 59.

Dr. Rose consulted Dr. Gabriel, an expert on MM at the Lineberger Comprehensive Cancer Center at UNC Hospitals in Chapel Hill. They proposed a course of treatment that we accepted immediately. We wanted to hit the disease as hard as we could.

We found Dr. Gabriel to be a brilliant scientist in addition to being a

17

caring doctor and a good teacher. His explanation of what we had and what we faced was detailed and elaborate, but very easy to understand.

He recommended a transplant within one year since that gave us the best opportunity of beating the monster disease that had overtaken Ambrose's body.

We agreed to plans for a transplant using Ambrose's stem cells rather than a donor's. To prepare Ambrose for the procedure, Dr. Rose would put him in the hospital four times for four days each.

During those hospital stays, Ambrose would be given three chemo drugs in a combination called VAD. (For those who want to know, VAD is a combination of vincristine, adriamycin, and dexamethasone or methylprednisolone.)

Ambrose became a familiar face on Rex Hospital's 5 West where one orderly said, "We have more fun on 5 West." His humor was a welcome breeze in the midst of so much hardship and pain.

The nurses who cared for Ambrose were another welcome addition to the team. We shared stories, experiences, and concerns with each other. They became part of our new family.

We came to realize that while undergoing treatment for a serious illness, you often make new friends both among the medical staff and other patients. We became closer with two families in our church. The husbands were also on the cancer floor undergoing treatment. We visited each other and lifted each other up in prayer. Unfortunately, both men later died.

One of the nurses slipped Ambrose hazelnut coffee when he awakened about 5 a.m. Otherwise, he would have had to suffer with instant coffee, which he just doesn't like.

The nurses would encourage his daily habit of exercising by taking long walks around the floor dragging his IV pole behind him. He couldn't leave the floor because he was taking chemo, and he couldn't get near other patients.

Ambrose named his IV pole "Clara Bell" for some reason. "Come on, Clara Bell, let's take a stroll," nurses would hear him say.

You notice that Ambrose found humor amidst his battle with cancer. His positive, can-do attitude was catching. People commented on his positive outlook. It kept the family in a great frame of mind.

Throughout the battle Ambrose became an inspiration to others. Dr. Billy F. Seate, our pastor at North Raleigh United Methodist Church, commented that Ambrose was a hero to some in the congregation. Others said he was their star, and doctors commented on his positive attitude and what a help this was to his recovery.

And we had our role models, too. One was Jim Cheek, a member of our church who had nine bouts with recurring cancer. Jim was one of the most cheerful people we had ever met and a big inspiration to Ambrose.

"Do what you've got to do and keep on trucking," he would tell Ambrose during their many conversations. Jim and Ambrose developed the mantra for dealing with a serious illness. It was based on trust in your doctors, the treatment plan, the body's ability to heal itself, and God's love.

In preparation for the SCT, we were contacted by the office of Betty Hinshaw, bone marrow transplant coordinator at UNC Hospitals.

Ambrose was alone at home when the first call came. He said all apprehension about the transplant just melted during that initial conversation. He said he felt like a member of the family was going to guide him through the SCT.

Betty was with us every step of the way. It is very comforting to have someone on the inside to help overcome obstacles when you are facing a very serious medical procedure.

Betty made appointments for us and made sure we were where we should be at the appointed time and that the doctors and other medical staff were there, too.

Betty gave us a calendar with everything we were to do at UNC written in on the appropriate date, including the proposed date of the SCT. She answered questions and provided reading material.

We also got tremendous support from Deborah Tucker of United

HealthCare (UHC), the AP's insurance carrier. She was UHC's transplant case manager.

Deb mailed Ambrose and me a packet of information about the transplant and the role of the caregiver. Deb called regularly during the treatment and was always available to help with insurance matters, of which there were few.

Ambrose's hospitalization in Chapel Hill for the SCT was sidetracked on three occasions by infections. His body just didn't like the double lumen catheter placed in his chest to receive the chemo.

Twice Ambrose spiked a fever of more than 101.5 degrees and was hospitalized in Raleigh. He had two more infections at UNC Hospitals, one on the day he was to begin treatment to harvest stem cells for the transplant. That delayed the process. The first catheter was removed after the infection was treated and the second, the day he completed a round of antibiotics after the transplant.

Ambrose and I were frustrated by the delays but were encouraged by some good reports we had gotten from blood work.

In July, the blood work report showed that the number of plasma cells in his bone marrow had dropped from 90 percent to 10 percent. The level of IgA plasma protein had dropped from 4,234 on February 18 to 567 on July 8. There was a faint band of paraprotein that the lab said wasn't worth pursuing.

The IMF pamphlet explains that the malignant plasma cells produce monoclonal immunoglobulins that appear as monoclonal "spikes" in the serum and/or urine.

Dr. Rose, sitting in Ambrose's hospital room discussing the report, wrote "normal" on his chart.

"I bet you are in a remission," he commented.

Ambrose said that was a fine birthday present. Since that day was Ambrose's birthday, I planned a surprise party that night in the wing's family room.

Although the word normal was used, we knew we needed the transplant to make sure we hit the cancer as hard as we could. MM is a sneaky disease.

It appeared we were in fine shape for the SCT. Ambrose had an excellent attitude, the four rounds of VAD had well prepared his body based on data from the blood tests, and we had a strong support system.

Our plans were made:

- We would close our house and move to Chapel Hill for the SCT, which could take up to three months.
- Our little Sheltie, Holly, would stay with our son Chris and his wife Kristy who lived near Chapel Hill.
- I would stay with my brother, Fred; Chris and Kristy; or Fred's former wife, Ann Henley. They all lived in or near Chapel Hill.
- I would stay with Ambrose during the day (9 a.m. to 6 p.m.) and then get some rest while the nurses cared for the sleeping patient.
- Friends would keep in touch in case we needed anything.
- We set up a telephone tree to keep everyone posted on developments. This would cut down on the number of phone calls both of us would have to make. Ambrose could take and make calls from his room, but we knew he would be resting or having treatment most of the time.
- Friends and family could visit his room. Anyone coming from outside the hospital would have to wash his or her hands for three minutes before entering. Those with sickness or colds were not allowed since Ambrose's immune system would be compromised or nonexistent much of the time.
- We made arrangements for Dr. Seate to visit regularly and for the prayer chain to keep lifting up Ambrose, our family, and me.
- Ambrose and I were comfortable with what was scheduled to happen and were prepared for the unexpected that could

happen during the SCT. We had spent a long weekend at the beach in early June discussing possibilities. We both knew that Ambrose could die during the transplant. We put our trust in God and did what we had to do.

We were ready. Boy, were we ready.

FOUR

AMBROSE: Alice didn't want to attend the meeting in the Research Triangle Park, but she was chosen to represent her school, Butner-Stem Elementary. Attendance was a must; there was no getting out of it.

She left school at 11:30 a.m., which would allow time for a comfortable drive directly to the RTP and for grabbing lunch along the way. She made it just south of Butner to the intersection of Cash Road and Old Weaver Trail in northern Wake County.

The police recorded the time of the accident involving a truck and an automobile at 11:39 a.m. Alice was knocked unconscious and suffered other serious injuries from the impact just in front of the driver's door.

The loving caregivers immediately began to envelop Alice.

David Wheeley, who lived near the scene, brought a cloth for Alice's forehead and a pillow for her head while his wife called 9-1-1. He turned off the car's engine. Authorities felt that in her serious condition, Alice needed to be taken to the hospital by helicopter ambulance.

The rescue squad cut Alice from the car and helped put her on the helicopter from Duke Medical Center in nearby Durham.

Authorities didn't immediately know her name. She was listed as Jane Doe upon arrival at Duke.

We were told later by doctors that the quick action to get a helicopter and the treatment provided during the flight from northern Wake County to Duke made a critical difference in Alice's recovery.

Internal bleeding and swelling of the brain are major concerns in severe closed head injuries. Alice had a bruise on the left side of her brain but no major swelling. She became one of 700,000 people, according to the National Head Injury Foundation, to be hospitalized annually because of a head injury.

Emergency room (ER) doctors found that Alice also had a bruised lung and had broken her clavicle, two ribs, her pelvis, and the tibia in her left leg. Small shards of glass punctured the left side of her face and her left hand and arm.

Officers located Alice's identification in the car's debris. A trooper drove to our home 25 minutes away. I was at work. A neighbor told him where to contact me.

It was a chilling feeling to hear those words on the phone during a busy news day: "Mr. Dudley, this is Trooper _____ of the North Carolina Highway Patrol ..."

I knew it wasn't good news because the route Alice traveled each day from North Raleigh to Butner was a dangerous, heavily traveled two-lane road. Frequently drivers showed great impatience at the many no-passing zones.

Alice had avoided a major accident a few weeks earlier by swerving onto the shoulder to miss a head-on collision with a large truck passing over a hill.

She was fortunate that time. This time tragedy struck.

The officer told me on the phone that Alice was taken to Duke. He didn't know if she was alive, but he knew her condition was serious.

I was calm during my transplant, but this shook me to the core. It was the start of a long period of uneasiness. My darling wife of 34 years was in danger.

I told the people at my office what I knew and said I didn't feel it was safe for me to drive the 23 miles from Raleigh to Durham. Sue Wilson, my dedicated news editor, said she would take me.

As we headed for Durham, I told Sue I was comforted by the fact that Alice and I had a practice of saying "I love you" as the last thing we told each other upon parting in the morning.

If she died, I knew "I love you" were the last words she had heard from me and that those wonderful words were the last I had heard from her lips.

We prayed in the car as we drove. I also either called or made arrangements for others to call members of the immediate family and close friends.

It was time for loved ones and caregivers to gather around. Family, friends, Alice's coworkers, and our pastor soon were in the ER waiting room at Duke.

Our son Greg was the tower of strength. He was such a comfort to others and me. Many commented later that Greg's cool demeanor was a godsend.

The ER doctor told those who first arrived that Alice was alive but in a deep coma, probably Rancho 2 level, one above a vegetable.

The Rancho Los Amigos Levels of Cognitive Function are as follows:

I. No Response: Patient appears to be in a deep sleep and is unresponsive to stimuli.

II. Generalized Response: Patient reacts inconsistently and nonpurposefully to stimuli in a nonspecific manner. Reflexes are limited and often the same, regardless of stimuli presented.

III. Localized Response: Patient responses are specific but inconsistent, and are directly related to the type of stimulus presented, such as turning head toward a sound or focusing on a presented object. He may follow simple commands in an inconsistent and delayed manner.

IV. Confused-Agitated: Patient is in a heightened state of activity and severely confused, disoriented, and unaware of present events. His behavior is frequently bizarre and inappropriate to his immediate environment. He is unable to perform self-care. If not physically disabled, he may perform automatic motor activities such as sitting, reaching and walking as part of his agitated state, but not necessarily as a purposeful act.

v. Confused-Inappropriate, Non-Agitated: Patient appears alert and responds to simple commands. More complex commands, however, produce responses that are nonpurposeful and random. The patient may show some agitated behavior it is in response to external stimuli rather than internal confusion. The patient is highly distractible and generally has difficulty in learning new information. He can manage self-care activities with assistance. His memory is impaired and verbalization is often inappropriate.

vi. Confused-Appropriate: Patient shows goal-directed behavior, but relies on cueing for direction. He can relearn old skills such as activities of daily living, but memory problems interfere with new learning. He has a beginning awareness of self and others.

vii. Automatic-Appropriate: Patient goes through daily routine automatically, but is robot-like with appropriate behavior and minimal confusion. He has shallow recall of activities, and superficial awareness of, but lack of insight to, his condition. He requires at least minimal supervision because judgment, problem solving, and planning skills are impaired.

viii. Purposeful-Appropriate: Patient is alert and oriented, and is able to recall and integrate past and recent events. He can learn new activities and continue in home and living skills, though deficits in stress tolerance, judgment, abstract reasoning, social, emotional, and intellectual capacities may persist.

The Duke doctors concentrated on the primary issue—the brain—and worried about caring for the other injuries later. We are convinced this was crucial in saving Alice's life and heading her on the road to some level of recovery.

There were many battles in the years ahead, but we had won the first one thanks to the love that immediately circled around Alice.

Alice's body began to heal although she was not aware of anything from the moments before the accident until she came out of the coma three weeks later. She remembered nothing about the time in the coma.

We kept a diary of the major mileposts in that recovery. I will walk through the highlights of that record and include some explanatory comments.

April 26: The traffic accident. Alice is flown to Duke, treated in the ER, and moved to the Intensive Care Unit (ICU).

May 7: Alice is moved from ICU to the step-down unit, into a private room, after doctors cleared up gram-positive, gram-negative, and staph infections that had settled in one of her lungs. It took three days of requests to get sutures removed from her hand and face. The caring community included Alice's niece's husband, Graham Snyder, who was about to graduate from UNC Medical School. It was a note from Graham that got the stitches removed. Another infection needed to be treated.

We found out how important it is for *all* members of the caring community to take the initiative to ask questions and push for treatment when it appears overlooked. While I was the primary caregiver for Alice, her sister Jane, brother Fred, Graham, and sons Chris and Greg and their wives were key players. Chris had to find a resident doctor late at night once to get more frequent suctioning of Alice's trachea tube, even though we had requested it several times during the day. We feel caregivers need to be always on guard and watching out for the patient.

May 10: Alice's birthday. Her breathing is labored with mucus in the lungs. Hard to get a straight answer from doctors and nurses as to why so many alarms are sounding from the equipment attached to Alice. The alarms diminished after more suctioning.

Once Alice's condition stabilized, we wanted to move her to a rehab hospital in Raleigh. Dr. Patrick O'Brien, with the advice of our friend Dr. Ted Kunstling, had established a first-class facility at Wake Medical Center.

A representative from WakeMed Rehab evaluated Alice. The labored breathing caused concern for the move.

A group of friends from her school brought a birthday cake and sang "Happy Birthday." It was beautiful. We wish Alice could have heard it. Some medical types told us that a person in a coma can hear what is going on and will recall much of it when they awake. That may be, but Alice didn't remember a thing. Children from Alice's school had sent a tape of messages to their counselor. They also drew pictures and made posters wishing her good health.

May 11: Breathing much better. Chest x-ray looked good. Alice is resting much more comfortably. Physical therapists put on a foot brace and left orders for it to be changed from one foot to the other every two hours when she was turned in the bed. We left a question for the doctors about whether the sutures from the operation to set the broken tibia needed to be removed.

May 12: Nurses turning Alice and changing her foot brace every couple of hours. Doctor checks feeding PEG (percutaneous enteral gastrostomy) tube in her stomach and says it is okay. He says the chest x-rays are consistently looking better. WakeMed says transfer delayed because of labored breathing. Nurse to remind doctor to remove stitches from the April 28 operation.

At 9 p.m. Chris and his wife, Kristy, made this entry in the diary:

"Great news! The nurse, Kris, and Chris went to turn Alice on her side and Alice opened her eyes. Since Kristy wasn't turning, she got very close to Alice's face. We are sure she focused! Also moving right hand and right leg a lot. Chris asked her to move her hand. She did. Then he held her hand and asked her to squeeze. She squeezed!!! Breathing much better. Also opened eyes again, especially right eye on her own part way for about 45 seconds. Yeah! Here's to wonderful steps of progress for Alice!"

At this point, some consider Alice out of the coma; others say she must do something consistently to be out. Anyway, it was great news.

May 13: Stitches in leg removed. Alice is beginning to be sweaty and move around more. The nurses call it "storming" a part of the healing process in a brain injury. It is slang for activities of head injury patients and probably meant she was moving from Ranchos 2 to 3. Alice is biting her lower lip, and the nurse gives her a mouth guard. WakeMed Rehab reevaluates Alice in hopes of finding some response from her. We told of Alice coughing on command and squeezing hands and the eye contact. WakeMed won't take a patient unless the doctors feel they can help the person. Otherwise the person would go to a rest home. That afternoon when the nurses changed Alice's position, her eyes opened. I put eyeglasses on her and told her to blink her eyes if she could see me. She did, twice! Alice continues to open her eyes when turned.

More good news—Alice will be moved to WakeMed Rehab tomorrow.

May 14: Alice had a good night and looked comfortable. She arrived at WakeMed at 12:17 p.m. and was met by Dr. O'Brien. Three hours later Alice opened her eyes for 3 minutes and blinked three times in response to me. She also had a smile on her face.

The caring community continued to expand as nurses cleaned Alice and tended to a rash between her legs and therapists asked the family to create a book of family pictures to help Alice remember things and people from her past.

May 15: Nurses had to stop feeding Alice via tube because the PEG site at her abdomen was leaking.

May 16: Alice opened her eyes and tracked me. Obviously, she is improving because the level of comprehension is increasing. She focused on a picture of granddaughter Emily. I called Chris and Greg. Chris arrived first.

"Mama, if you love me blink your eyes," Chris asked.

She blinked twice. Then she opened her eyes and smiled at us.

Alice was back! Now, the months of rehab could begin.

May 17: PEG replaced. Alice smiles a lot. Progress continued daily with Alice being more alert and responsive.

May 26: Alice moved her mouth as if she would like to talk.

May 27: Collar around her neck was removed, and Alice was placed in a wheelchair.

May 28: Doppler studies showed a thrombosis (blood clot) in the upper left arm. It was treated with a blood thinner, and tests were conducted regularly. (Credit Graham with a good job of suspecting a blood clot, which are not always easy to spot.)

May 29: Trachea plugged at night to see if Alice could breathe on her own. She quickly showed she could.

June 3: Neuropsychologist reports Alice is more restless and probably is moving through Ranchos 3 to Ranchos 4.

June 4: Dr. O'Brien makes rounds and enters Alice's room with the usual cheerful "Good morning, Mrs. Dudley. How are you?" He didn't necessarily expect a response from the patient.

"I feel fine," Alice responded.

Those were her first words since the accident, and they were in the form of a sentence, which gave us all great hope.

A daily routine of speech, physical, and occupational therapy was begun. Family and friends were kept posted on progress through written weekly reports and daily comments from doctors, nurses, and therapists.

June 11: Alice is in Ranchos 5—trying to control her environment. Bones have healed to the place where doctors allowed her to stand up in preparation for trying to walk.

June 12: Alice talked about being in a coma and said she wanted to send a message to the members of North Raleigh United Methodist Church.

The message:

"I love you. I appreciate your support. I appreciate your continual prayers."

June 17: Started showing her sense of humor with nurses and staff. Since she still could not move on her own, Alice asked a nurse, "Who glued me to the bed?"

June 23: Started feeding herself.

June 25: Wrote her name.

June 26: Wrote a note to her Sunday school class.

As Alice could communicate more we found she had double vision, some back pain, and was very anxious.

July 9: Alice walked 30 feet with two assistants and a walker.

July 13: Alice is in Ranchos 6.

July 15: Alice starts eating with other patients.

July 20: The PEG is removed.

July 24: Alice gets a day pass to leave the hospital and be at home in preparation for discharge. The family gathered around, and we had a steak dinner that Alice enjoyed. She also enjoyed a nap on the couch.

July 30: Alice and I spent the night together at the rehab hospital's temporary living suite. This allowed us to get used to living alone again. A nurse was available one floor up to answer any questions.

Aug. 3: Alice is discharged and comes home with a pocketful of prescriptions.

The workload really picks up for the primary caregiver. But I love it! My dear Alice is home again.

FIVE

AMBROSE: When life hits the hard times, Alice and I have found in sixty-six years of living that a person must dig deeper into his or her being for strength. We found our faith provided the strength we needed for facing the struggles ahead. God is the ground of our being, as the theologian Paul Tillich said.

We and others we met in the walk toward recovery talked frequently about how hard it would be to deal with the daily heartaches without a deep, working relationship with God. We feel a mere casual acquaintance with God is not enough. The relationship needs to be renewed daily.

It was months after my diagnosis when Alice and I finally talked about the reality that I could die during the battle with cancer. Both of us had known the possibility from the beginning.

The days between February and June had been filled with chemo treatments, conferences with doctors, and one decision after another. Alice had continued to work, knowing she would have to be absent for three or four months when I had the transplant.

Life was hectic, and we had not taken the time to talk about the what-ifs. Our friends the Kunstlings let us use their beach place in early June of 1997.

I was weak from the chemo treatments, and my body was not fully cooperating, but I was at the beach. I had always been a beach person. I found I could do some of my best thinking walking slowly along the sandy coast letting the waves come near my feet. The steady rhythm of the waves is curative to my soul.

I looked out the top-floor window and saw the blue ocean and sandy beach beyond the front-row houses. It put me in the spirit to think and talk about the future. It wasn't that we had tried to avoid it in the past. It was that we just had not had "the talk."

"You know this thing could kill me," I said to Alice.

We talked and we talked. We realized we had met the enemy face-to-face and were very comfortable with the choices and decisions we had made.

With her usual counselor advice, Alice suggested we look at the future beyond the transplant and make some plans that we could hold on to. Our first promise was to take another trip to Bermuda, which both of us love.

During that weekend I took a hard look at my life, also. I did a lot of soul searching and talking with God. Alice had always told me my caustic sense of humor and somewhat gruff approach sometimes left a lot of hurt in my wake.

I decided to improve on some of the rough spots in my personality and to plan things I wanted to do.

The doctors say the day in the SCT when the patient gets a stem cell infusion is the beginning of the person's second life.

Using that as the guide, I sat at the beach cottage table and wrote out this list for

MY SECOND LIFE

- Show God's love to one person at a time by letting that person know he/she is the most important person at that moment. (Sometimes I looked past people and didn't really listen to them.)
- Spend quality time with Alice. (My work had been demanding in terms of long hours and many road trips. I needed to spend quality time with her and do some things we both enjoy, like traveling).
- Answer God's elective call to the lay or ordained ministry. (There was this urge deep within me to be a United Methodist minister. I

went through the candidacy program and was headed toward being a part-time local pastor when cancer sidetracked me. I needed to find another avenue for helping others and serving Him).

- Be patient. (Patience has never been my long suit.)
- Enjoy daily each experience, each person. (I wanted to appreciate people more for their assets rather than looking for deficits.)
- Recognize that I am a new person.
- Release the old self. (Get rid of all that junk I have been carrying around.)
- Use resources to do fun and fulfilling things. (Alice learned while studying Reality Therapy that one of the basic needs of life is to have fun.)
- Give more time to worthwhile projects like my work with older adults at the Sheets Day Care center at Edenton Street United Methodist Church.
- Recognize and appreciate more fully the significance and importance of the presence of God in everyday life.
- The second life is a kind of nirvana: Moving to a higher level and a fuller life.
- Be a pelican: He lives at the beach, spends his days flying up and down the coast looking for food, and is the biggest bird around. (The pelican is a symbol of being happy, fulfilled, and above the day's nuisances.)
- Let the Holy Spirit be my guide in all endeavors.
- Realize that the Second Life is a miracle from God that is to be used in His service. Thus this book.
- Witness for Him in everything I do for as long as I do it.

The list worked. It made me look beyond the present crisis and gave me something to anticipate. It was part of the positive attitude I took into the battle with cancer.

After Alice was injured, and once I found out she would be with me for a while longer, I did similar planning. When she came out of the coma, I told her some of my thinking. Our planning included things for the future like a trip abroad (Ireland first) and a cruise (around the Caribbean). Having something to look forward to helped in her recovery and mine.

Underlying our ability to face the reality of our situation is our faith. Many people have contributed to building our faith over the years. It is like our lives were a preparation for battle.

I can think of many examples and the advice of different people that contributed to our getting through the twin crises. There were a number of sermons by pastors over the years that came to mind in the midst of the struggles.

One that particularly stands out was a sermon preached by Pastor Robinson at Dilworth UMC in Charlotte. He was a tower of strength with a gift for preaching powerful sermons. He later died of cancer.

This particular sermon was included in a book of his sermons—*Happy ... If with My Latest Breath*—that his family published after his death on October 9, 1964. He had served more than thirty years in the ministry.

The sermon concerned those times when life reaches its most difficult points. Pastor Robinson said:

> Then, when one's faith faces that last extremity, when the worst comes to the worst, there's always the possibility that adversity can bring enrichment to one's personal life. I am aware that trouble makes some people bitter and cynical, but it may have the opposite effect. It may bring out in character all the fine qualities that have been dormant beneath the surface during the sunshine. We all know people who have learned in the flame some lesson that they failed to learn in the mildness of the sunshine.

The sermon impressed me when he gave it, and its message has stayed with me through the years. That is how we help each other. We never know when something we do will empower a person at his or her point of need, even if it is many years later.

Alice and I both dug deep in our being to call forth such gems as we continued the battle and looked at the reality of what had happened to us. We hoped we could use our difficult circumstances to be better people and better servants.

Then there were the treasures we found in reading. Somewhere I came across a work by Dr. Susan W. N. Ruach, Director of Conference Spiritual Leadership Development for the United Methodist General Board of Discipleship in Nashville, Tennessee, that took a new look at struggle. This poem was instrumental in helping me see our struggle from a different perspective and look at the future more hopefully. It goes:

— A NEW WAY OF STRUGGLING —

by Dr. Susan W. N. Ruach

To struggle used to be
to grab with both hands
and shake, twist, turn, push
and shove and not give in.

But wrest an answer from it all
as Jacob did a blessing.

There is another way to struggle
with an issue, a question—

Simply to jump off into the abyss
and find ourselves
floating...

falling...

tumbling...

being led slowly and gently,
but surely to the answers God has for us—
to watch the answers unfold before our eyes
and still be a part of the unfolding.
      But, oh! the trust necessary for this new way!
Not to be always reaching out for the old hand-holds.

I had that poem with me during the transplant and plotted the fall and rise of my white blood count with the words in her work. It fit. As the count fell and fell I saw myself tumbling and then watched the answers unfold.

The poem helped me deal with the reality of the situation.

During the uncertain days of Alice's coma, I recalled the new way I had learned to deal with the struggle. I never lost faith that she would come out of the coma and we would make that Caribbean cruise.

I didn't know if she would come back as she was before the accident. I didn't know what condition I would be in. But I was confident that hand in hand we could deal with the future.

SIX

"Behold, I make all things new."
Revelation 21:5

ALICE: My memory is somewhat impaired since my accident, but luckily I kept a diary during Ambrose's hospitalization. I will rely on it for the following description.

I will try not to be too technical, but I do need to tell a little about the process for a bone marrow transplant (BMT)/stem cell transplant (SCT). In Ambrose's case it technically was a peripheral blood stem cell transplant (PBSCT). We will refer to it as SCT.

After the rounds of VAD, Ambrose went to UNC Hospitals for preparation for the SCT. Transplant preparation involved doses of chemo to mobilize his system and shots at home to promote cell growth.

We had fun giving Ambrose two shots each night. We both are better patients than nurses. I would give the shot in the arm, and Ambrose would be responsible for the one in the calf. He wasn't very good and often hit a vein putting the needle in or pulling it out. This would leave a big bruise on his leg.

The next step was apheresis, which involved Ambrose lying in a bed for five hours while his blood ran through a machine that separated the different parts of the blood. The stem cells were collected, and the remainder was recirculated.

The process often takes five days and up to four hours each day. The goal is to collect about five million stem cells during the week.

My Ambrose showed his stuff in apheresis.

When we returned for the second day, the nurse said we could go home. We were surprised. Our first thought was that they had decided not to continue the process leading to a transplant. That would have been tragic since without an SCT Ambrose's life expectancy was only months. Our hearts sank.

But the nurse said just the opposite was the case. Ambrose had produced 14.1 million stem cells the first day. The blood bank director came to the waiting room to congratulate us. Ambrose had set a record! It was the first of two records he would set during the SCT at UNC.

We checked with Betty Hinshaw, the BMT coordinator, to make sure she agreed we had collected enough stems cells, which would be the source of life for Ambrose after the cells remaining in his body were killed. She said they had enough and we could enjoy a few days of rest before reporting to the hospital Sunday morning.

We have praised the Lord many times for the high stem cell count. We were told that his marrow must have been in good condition in order to produce cells like that.

Ambrose's cells were frozen for storage. We went home to relax for a few days. And we needed it. The whole process had been taxing on both of us. We enjoyed the few days off.

The actual SCT process uses a system of dates, starting with minus 5. That is the day the patient enters the hospital. The days are counted down to zero, the day of the "rescue." That is when the stem cells are returned to the patient. From then on it is day plus 1, plus 2, plus 3, and so on.

I need to explain one other technical point that will help in understanding the SCT.

The medical staff kept a close watch on Ambrose's blood counts, particularly the white cell count. Normally it is 4.5 to 11. The red blood count (hematocrit [hct]) is 41 to 53, and the platelet count 150 to 440. Each day's readings were posted on a board in Ambrose's hospital room.

A successful procedure would take the white count to as close to zero as possible. When the transplanted cells engraft, the count rises. We will pay attention only to the white count.

Rather than relying on my memory, I want to let you read my diary:

September 14 (-5 day) Ambrose entered the hospital. Chris helped us get up to the unit at UNC hospitals. (The "unit" is the bone marrow unit on the fifth floor near the UNC Burn Center.) Most of the first day was spent getting settled in, having the nurses take blood for lab reports, seeing the doctor, etc., etc. A six-hour saline solution was followed by a "lethal" dose of melphlan, the chemotherapy that is given as a part of this protocol.

We expect Ambrose to be quite ill in a week or so from this potent drug. It is supposed to do a job on his mouth and throat (where the body creates cells most often, making them more susceptible to pain). The doctors gave him kitral and decadron beforehand to prevent nausea. (*Comment from Ambrose*: Kitral is a wonder drug that tells the stomach and the brain to ignore the chemo. It worked!)

Ambrose's main doctor, Don Gabriel, is a first-rate hematologist/oncologist. His specialty is myeloma, and he is highly respected by those who work with him. He is off in-service duty in the transplant unit during September and October, but he stopped by Ambrose's room a number of times.

Dr. Joe Wiley, a pediatric hematologist/oncologist, is on duty in the BMT unit during September. He is very nice and sharp, as well. He is very knowledgeable about multiple myeloma. A "fellow" oncology student, Dr. Tom Hensing, will be working with Dr. Wiley this month. He had a good visit with us.

I am staying with Fred, my brother, who lives about seven minutes from the hospital. I got settled in about 12:30 p.m. and then went back to the "Big House," as Ambrose fondly calls the hospital. Greg and Beth, our older son and his wife, visited before Beth left for Colorado to see her new niece.

Ambrose and I often spoke of how fortunate we are to have four wonderful children—our two sons and their wives. We enjoy much love in our family. We think that helped Ambrose get through this nightmare.

Ambrose was doing well after his round of chemo, and I left just after 7 p.m.

September 15 (-4 day) Ambrose's blood counts were very good. It was ironic that his marrow is in good shape and his blood counts are good. All that will drastically change in order to prepare (clean out the cancer cells) for the transplant which will be Friday (0 day).

The combination of high-dose chemo and total body irradiation (TBI), which started today on a twice-a-day basis, will destroy his marrow to make room for his beautiful and abundant stem cells, currently stored in the blood bank.

The Bible verse in the *Upper Room* meditation for Sunday was:

> *"Be strong and of good courage; do not be frightened or dismayed,*
> *for the Lord your God is with you wherever you go."*
>
> *(Joshua 1:9)*

We must cling to this verse!

September 16 (-3 day) It is late. I am back at Fred's, and I'm tired. Ambrose's day wasn't as good as yesterday. He has had some nausea, but medications are plentiful to help relieve it. White count still very good. The Doppler studies from yesterday showed that he still has a blood clot that developed in his right shoulder with his first Hickman double lumen apheresis catheter, a line that goes into his artery.

A volunteer today massaged his sore back. He has a chronic pain in his shoulder.

Greg came by, and we attended a support group. It was very good. It was discouraging to talk with a woman whose husband has been in the hospital 41 days since his transplant, and he has had pneumonia and graft vs. host disease and isn't doing too well. He had a donor transplant (allogeneic) for leukemia. Ambrose's SCT is autologous because he will use his own cells.

Ambrose has been going twice a day for TBI. He likes the technicians, but I think all that radiation is taking a toll. He was very tired and sleepy. I went to dinner with younger son Chris and his wife, Kristy.

September 17 (-2 day) More TBI. I give support.

September 18 (-1 day) Tomorrow Ambrose gets his cells back. He'll probably sleep right through the procedure as tired as he is now.

I didn't write yesterday. I was too busy being entertained. So many wonderful people care for us, and we feel so blessed. I packed up and left Fred's temporarily as he is leaving on a trip and I didn't want to stay alone in his home in the woods. I am staying at Ann Henley's home for a few days. She and Fred both live within minutes of the hospital, and both have very nice accommodations for me.

Went to the Loop for grilled veggie pizza with June Cross (who taught music at Butner-Stem elementary school where I am a guidance counselor) yesterday. Ambrose and I both enjoyed seeing her. She's such a dear person to me.

Last night, Chris took Greg and me to meet a friend for dinner at Spankey's. Very good to see all of them. (*Note from Ambrose*: You notice how Alice is taking care of herself and enjoying dining with friends. It is very important for the caregiver to enjoy a life outside the hospital. Also, Alice is enjoying Chapel Hill eateries while I was trying to down hospital food and cold coffee from plastic cups, which took its toll on this particular morning.)

Today, Ambrose has gotten increasingly weaker and wants to sleep most of the time. He threw up a little bit this morning (after trying to drink coffee from a plastic cup), but the antinausea meds have been slightly adjusted and he is feeling a little better, I think. He ate chicken soup for lunch and a couple of crackers.

Yesterday, I went down to radiation with him and watched the technicians do the TBI. It was interesting, and he doesn't seem to mind it. Ambrose is placed in a room alone. He is sitting on a device that resembles a wooden horse with a comfortable seat. He cannot move for twenty minutes. He is radiated on one side and then on the other for ten minutes each. There is some sort of plate that protects his brain from getting too much radiation. His lethargy and nausea are coming from the radiation. The main effect from the chemo should hit hard in a few days.

The doctors are pleased he is progressing normally. His white count hit 100 yesterday and 90 today. I feel good about things so far. Even though this is scary, it is very interesting. We are hoping for an early engraftment of the stem cells. It generally takes seven to fifteen days, but the record-breaking stem cell collection may help him have an early engraftment.

I am glad I am here for Ambrose. He loves having me here, but he doesn't feel like making conversation.

September 19 (0 day) This is the big day.

We are looking forward to "a whole new life" as Reynolds Price said in his book about his battle with cancer.

Ambrose has taped a number of Bible verses, poems, and sayings on his wall where he could see them each day. The writings give him support.

The one from Revelation was very appropriate for today.

"Behold, I make all things new." (Rev. 21:5)

We are so very excited about the events of this morning. Lee from the blood lab came up with Ambrose's "life" and all the machinery needed for the infusion. She prepared the bags of cells to be re-infused. The stem cells were frozen. She warmed the cells and gave them to Amy, Ambrose's wonderful nurse today. Amy put the cells into a huge syringe and put that into the central line.

The actual transplant started at 10:15 a.m. and was complete by 11 a.m. It is called "the rescue" for good reason.

The process is all very simple considering the very real and dramatic impact it has on our lives! It's not an operation. One doesn't even leave the room, but wonderful new life is infused into Ambrose's body to replace the marrow that has been destroyed by chemotherapy and radiation. He was glad to have his last radiation treatment yesterday afternoon.

Our pastor, Dr. Billy Seate, came by early for the "rescue" procedure. He led us all in a prayer just before the stem cells were returned to Ambrose. Ambrose is now reading aloud Bible verses of praise. We are both very excited and grateful. It was a touching moment. One of the nurses had tears in her eyes.

His white count is 0.8.

September 20 (+1 day) Ambrose's white count is most unusual and unexpected. It is 9.5—in the normal range. The doctors and nurses would have expected it to continue dropping until it bottomed out below 0.1.

At first, the doctors thought the lab had made an error, but it was rechecked and still read 9.5. The doctor on call now feels that is a fluke—sort of a last-ditch rally before the counts bottom out. The nurses are very surprised that the count is so high. Of course, Ambrose's stem cell collection during apheresis was surprising, too.

Now the question is whether the white count on Day +1 is just a fluke or the transplant miraculously engrafted and started producing new cells. Tomorrow's count will tell.

Typically, Ambrose would be entering into the lowest period now for one to two weeks. The marrow has been destroyed by chemo and radiation, and the new cells would not have engrafted.

Even if this count today is a last hurrah before the fall, we are still hopeful that the good stem cell collection will help with an early engraftment.

The Lord is really in all of this no matter how it goes. Ambrose and I had a good talk about it this morning. We are very excited and hopeful. Ambrose continues to have a very, very positive attitude about life even though he feels rotten. This is one of the things I love about him. His positive attitude is an inspiration to all of us, in and out of the hospital.

September 21 (+2 day) The blood counts:

White	2.4
Red	8.9
Platelets	204

So the white count did take a considerable dip today. Eileen Powell, the nurse practitioner who is so much a part of the UNC BMT program, and the physician on duty while Dr. Wiley was away paid a visit. They feel good about Ambrose's condition and told us to expect him not to feel well this week as the counts continue to fall.

Eileen said yesterday's high white count was probably the result of the effect of growth factor shots on some remaining marrow that was still lingering around.

Ambrose is low today, psychologically and physically. He ate some breakfast and felt fairly well for a while but is sinking as the day goes on. He doesn't want to eat or drink.

Amy, his overnight nurse this weekend, said it was OK because he is getting fluid through his IV.

A number of friends stopped by to visit. Kristy and Chris and their friend C. R. also visited. I took them all out for BBQ. BBQ is not on my late-night diet usually, but it was fun being all together. Beth and Greg had been by earlier in the day.

I hope Ambrose won't be too sick this week, but it is pretty par for the course, we are told.

September 22 (day +3) Ambrose's white count is 0.2. He is very weak, but in wonderful spirits. He is dressed and has eaten oatmeal and juice for breakfast. He had half a pimento cheese sandwich and V-8 juice that I brought him for lunch.

The prophets of "gloom and doom" constantly preached at us about how sick he is going to be. How sore his mouth will be, how pitifully his GI tract will behave, tube feedings, infections, and so on. They predicted it could be fourteen days before he engrafted. All I can say is it is Day +3 and his white count is nearly nonexistent and he is doing fine, but is tired.

He may hit a lower low, or this may be it. His white count will drop further, and beyond that we don't know.

We really appreciate Dr. Wiley. He has returned from a weekend visit to his ailing father. He was very upbeat about Ambrose's condition. He said he is doing much better than one would typically do at this time. He said to expect a few low days. Then when his count starts coming back, he will really take off very quickly. Dr. Wiley is very optimistic. He thinks because of his super-duper stem cells, he will do very well. Dr. Wiley says there are a number of favorable conditions all working together.

(*Comments from Ambrose*: Notice the difference between the doom and gloom set who told me that it would be ten to fourteen days before I engrafted and how I would feel horrible and Dr. Wiley's words of encouragement. Before he left for the weekend, Dr. Wiley had given me a pep talk about how I was doing and predicted I could set an adult record by engrafting on Day +6. We knew that possibility was far out, but his encouragement gave me the pickup I needed. Especially when twenty minutes later Nurse Gloom came into the room with the "you are going to feel terrible for two weeks" routine. Three years after the SCT I was asked to talk with second-year med students at UNC on occasion. I used this example to show how their upbeat approach, while not misleading a patient, can be a real plus. Those caring for the patient need to be sensitive to how their attitude affects the patient and his or her family.)

Ambrose received two bags of blood (a red cell concentrate) since his hemoglobin and hct were low. The transfusions should give him a little more zip.

I feel very upbeat today about Ambrose's condition. I think he will do well. This whole thing is a spiritual journey for both of us. Ambrose's attitude since learning in February he had cancer has been upbeat and extremely positive. He has touched many lives.

I went to dinner at the Rathskeller with our friends Ted and Frances Kunstling.

September 23 (Day +4) Ambrose is very weak today. His white count hit 0.1, and he had a low-grade fever. Ambrose felt well enough to ride his stationary bike for ten minutes. Patients are encouraged to ride the bike daily to keep muscles in shape. Sores in his mouth are a problem, but there is not much pain. He has no appetite most of the time. He does like friend Sara Nichol's coffee cake, and I called Sara to make another one.

I have moved back to Fred's and went there to do some laundry. Ambrose was unsettled at night by a nurse who talked gloom and doom. He called me to get some comforting words. I told him just to remember all the good things Dr. Wiley had said and reminded him that he is looking for an early engraftment. I hope he won't be disappointed. Someone told me she doesn't expect him to engraft before Day +10 because the radiation prevents early engraftment. The medical person said radiation also was why he was slow to drop his counts. Anyway, this is one view. It will be interesting to see when his counts do come back up. Ambrose is shooting for Day +6, and I am saying Day +7. Either of these would be terrific.

September 24 (Day +5) A gloomy, rainy day outside. Ambrose's counts are even lower. He is really not in much pain. He is just low and feels useless. He told someone he was "bottom fishing." He wants his counts to go up tomorrow to set a record for early engraftment by an adult. Dr. Wiley continues to be his cheerful self and keeps reminding Ambrose of how far he will go up when his cells take off. Wiley said he was going to Toronto for a conference and he was sure Ambrose would be engrafted by the time he returned on Sunday (Day +9). Ambrose said we should record this as "just another day of waiting at the bottom." Ironically, his appetite is some better today. I read a lot of scripture to Ambrose before I left for the night. The knowledge of God's love is really sustaining him.

Ambrose drew strength from the writing "Footprints" by Margaret Fishback Powers.

Ambrose felt like he was being carried through the SCT by the Lord.

September 25 (Day +6) His counts are still down and Ambrose realized he had missed his goal for engrafting today. But he is very upbeat. He continues to do fine. I read his meditation books to him and sang a hymn. Dr. Gabriel popped in, just back from Denmark. He had some interesting comments, and, as always, we felt better after having been with him. We always learn from him. He was sweet to drop by when he wasn't on duty this month. I went to lunch with a friend, and Ambrose took another nap. It is another day of "bottom fishing" for Ambrose.

SEVEN

ALICE:

September 26 (Day +7) "I have good news today!" exclaimed the nurse as she burst through the door to write on the board the latest blood count numbers.

"Your white count is 0.2," she said.

Ambrose let out a shout of joy.

He had engrafted on Day +7. We were heading back to health just as Dr. Wiley had predicted.

Ambrose called me at Fred's with the good news and I called the boys. We said a prayer of thanks on the phone.

They did another count later in the day and the white count had doubled.

September 27 (Day +8) Ambrose's white count was 1.7. That is terrific. Drs. Hensing and Wiley are very, very pleased with his progress. Ambrose, of course, feels much better and is no longer nauseated. He ate eggs and bacon for breakfast and a hamburger for lunch.

Dr. Wiley, who had just returned from Toronto, predicted we'd be out of the hospital by next weekend. He said I didn't need to do anything extraordinary to prepare the house for Ambrose's homecoming. I needed to have the rugs cleaned and remove all the houseplants or put the plants in a room Ambrose won't use. He also exiled our dog Holly for a while longer.

I went to lunch at 411 West with friends Anna and Ben Neimitz, who own the cottage next to ours in the mountains of Ashe County. They live in Chapel Hill.

Everyone has been so nice to me. Ambrose has received many, many cards and balloons and calls. He can't receive flowers. Support has been abundant from friends, colleagues, church members, neighbors and others. We are most grateful with this and with Ambrose's progress. He is really doing extraordinarily well.

I look at all the IVs (medication dripped into his body) he is receiving and all the attention he gets from nurses and wonder how I can possibly handle all this in a week or so. Hopefully, he won't be needing as much. I am going to Raleigh tonight to begin getting the house cleaned up before my husband comes home!

September 29 (Day +10) Sunday was another day of healing. This morning Ambrose's blood counts were:

> White 12.8
>
> Hemoglobin 10.8
>
> Hematocrit 29.3
>
> Platelets 50

When Beth and Greg were visiting they accompanied Ambrose on his first walk outside his room. He donned a face mask and went strolling. He enjoyed being out of the room a lot.

Missing the first walk made me feel as though I'd missed my baby's first steps. I have been with Ambrose about ten or more hours each day and I hated to be away from him. I really worked in Raleigh, mostly dealing with clutter, my nemesis, and arrived back in Chapel Hill exhausted. It was a wonderful feeling being at home enjoying the kitchen we had remodeled just before the transplant, the beautiful flowers and the vibrant green grass refreshed by the recent rains. I can hardly wait to drive Ambrose home. I am a little scared, too, if the truth be known.

Doctors were concerned about Ambrose not drinking enough liquids. A night nurse told Ambrose to try Gatorade for taste and an instant breakfast for substance. It worked. The tube feedings were reduced in volume with the idea of weaning him. He tried to eat too many solids and got upset. A nurse told him to think of his GI tract as that of a baby's and take liquids first and go slowly with solids.

I saw Dr. Gabriel in the afternoon. He is pleased with how Ambrose is doing. He gave me a sober reminder though of how extremely difficult this disease is. Our primary focus these days has been to come back from the onslaught of the conditioning and the transplant. We haven't focused on the cancer. How I pray he has a CR, a complete response.

Dr. Gabriel said the worst-case scenario would be that the SCT gives him some time, and there are promising treatments being developed. Of course, we are hoping and expecting the best case. I can't help but think that this good response—the good cells and all that—and his quick engraftment and how quickly his white count has gone up—that all this is an indication of how he'll do with the Big C.

September 30 (Day +11) I am attending a support group that I attended last Tuesday and the one before. The other caregivers who come all seem to be from the allogeneic (donor stem cells) side of the BMT unit and their loved ones are experiencing so many more problems than Ambrose is. I am so grateful he is doing well.

October 4 (Day +15) I have been a bad girl. I haven't written for days and so much has happened. Ambrose has continued to improve! On Day +12 Dr. Hensing said he might be discharged Friday (Day +14). Dr. Wiley came by Tuesday evening on his final visit as he goes off inpatient rotation at the end of September. He is very pleased with how Ambrose has done and has very complimentary things to say about both of us and how much he has enjoyed us.

Ambrose's optimistic spirit has cheered up everyone and all seem to think it has contributed to his doing so well. As Ambrose says, "So far this hasn't been nearly as bad as was advertised."

Anyway, Wiley told us that the discharge probably would be Friday or Saturday. The only thing keeping him is for him to increase his intake of fluids. The tube feeding was discontinued Tuesday p.m.

We are both so grateful for Joe Wiley and told him how much he lifted our spirits. I went to dinner with Kristy and Chris at 411 West to celebrate. Ambrose dined on hospital food.

With the news that Ambrose was coming home in two or three days, I went to Raleigh on Wednesday (Day +12). My friend June Cross met me there to help get the house in order for the patient. June is really a worker. She is an outstanding example of how a friend can be a great caregiver: drop everything you are doing and come when the person needs you.

The carpet cleaners met us at the house and I had them steam clean most of the carpet. I saved the guest room as a dumping ground for all my clutter, boxes and stuff I otherwise didn't know what to do with.

There are still boxes in the living room from the kitchen remodeling project that was completed a week before we left the house. I will get to those boxes at my leisure. Ambrose convinced me there was no rush because he wasn't going in there and the doctors have said we can keep houseplants in one room. We also had the sofa and upholstered chair cleaned. The installer showed up and put up the new mini blinds in the kitchen, breakfast room and bathroom. We had ordered the blinds before the transplant.

I was rather proud of myself for getting all of this organized and also grateful that it all came together for me. We can't have people in and out cleaning and installing with Ambrose home.

After June and the service people left, I worked into the night cleaning, etc. In the morning, I washed the noncarpeted floors. I had an appointment with my doctor to do a blood pressure check. The new medicine I am on doesn't seem to be doing as good a job as the previous one did, but I couldn't tolerate that bad cough it gave me.

My doctor, Jane Smith, and her nurse were thrilled that Ambrose was doing so well. Dr. Smith asked me to stay on the medication for six more weeks.

I returned to Chapel Hill to get my husband!

Dr. Tom Shea, head of the BMT program at UNC, followed Dr. Wiley in the unit. He had come by Wednesday evening and told Ambrose he would be discharged on Thursday (Day +13)! The nurse had tipped me Wednesday morning that there was scuttlebutt that he would leave earlier than previously thought. So I was prepared.

It really is astonishing that Ambrose would be released on Day +13, not even three weeks after he arrived at the hospital.

Dr. Karen Albritton, an oncology fellow we had known for a couple of months, said Ambrose might be the first adult to leave the unit that quickly.

"We've had children to leave that soon, but I'm not aware of any other adults!" she said.

Eileen Powell later confirmed that it was a record for an adult.

So my Ambrose had set two records at UNC—number of stems cells given the first day of apheresis and the earliest date for discharge of an adult after an SCT. He tied the record for adult engraftment.

My body ached from all the work I did in Raleigh, but we were both excited about going home! Ambrose still has been eating very little at a time and he was looking forward to going home, sitting in his chair and drinking soup out of a ceramic mug.

The presentation of the meal had a lot to do with the turnoff Ambrose felt about the hospital's food. We talked to Dr. Wiley and the nutritionist about this. We have all heard about studies aimed at making food more appealing to BMT patients.

Discharge took a while. I got back from Raleigh in plenty of time to wait. The nurse showed me how to change the new type of dressing for Ambrose's central line (catheter). That was about it. Ambrose is going home with just a few medicines. Usually, a patient leaves the BMT unit with many medications. We have been so very, very fortunate!

Ambrose's blood count numbers were impressive. His white count went from 1.7 on Day +8 to 8.6 on Day +9 to 12.8 on Day +10. The day we went home the white count had settled to 8.2, quite normal. His platelets were at 99 and hemoglobin at between 10 and 11. So he had to be careful.

During the nineteen days in the hospital, Ambrose didn't develop an infection or have any real complications. Complications, infections and fever are the norm, so he was exceptionally lucky. We still have a couple of months (through Day +60) when he will be very, very vulnerable and could become ill. So we don't want to be cocky about the fact that he hasn't been ill yet.

At this point, I quit keeping a diary and devoted my energy to caring for my husband.

Ambrose would return to UNC Hospitals three times a week for checkups for a while.

In fact, he got to return to UNC Hospitals as an inpatient the next week. Ambrose developed a gram-negative, gram-positive infection from the catheter and had to be hospitalized.

It was the fourth infection he had gotten since May from the catheter. The first line had been removed after three infections. This one came out after he had completed his antibiotic drip. We were delighted to get rid of that thing.

One doctor told us, "Those things are always trouble." Ambrose' body just didn't like that foreign object.

Dr. Gabriel allowed our Sheltie, Holly, to return home after Day +60. After Day +100, he said, Ambrose could do what he felt like doing.

Ambrose has visited either Dr. Gabriel or Dr. Rose every three months for blood tests and checkups. A biopsy was done of his bone marrow at least once a year for seven years.

For three years after the SCT there was a faint band of paraprotein reported by the lab. It disappeared in August 2000. In February 2001 we got the following report on the latest biopsy from Dr. Gabriel in an e-mail:

"No paraprotein detectable and < 3% plasma cells … = CR"

That was the outstanding news we had been seeking since the diagnosis of MM in February 1997.

The initial tests showed that 90 percent of Ambrose's bone marrow was sheets of plasma cells. Four years later that number was reduced to less than 3 percent.

A complete response (CR) is the hoped-for outcome of an SCT/BMT.

We were delighted, but realized there was no cure for MM. There is a tremendous amount of hope, however.

EIGHT

… A cheerful heart has a continual feast.
Proverbs 15:15

And the peace of God, which passes all understanding,
will keep your hearts and your minds in Christ Jesus.
Philippians 4:7

AMBROSE: I never really thought of myself as a positive person. In fact, I thought I had a pretty negative outlook on life. I had the view of life as a glass half empty and believed I didn't have much to offer. I was sure whatever I achieved in life was a gift and not deserved.

This probably came from my childhood (therapists like for you to use that as an excuse). My mother seemed to have passed along to me her insecurities. She became emotionally upset when my father would not come through the door in the evening at the exact minute she expected.

An emotionally upset mother can have a big impact on a small child, especially if he is growing up with an inferiority complex. I was tearful through many of the years I was in elementary school and the teachers had to give me lots of tender loving care.

I began to grow out of that in high school but had a relapse in college when I had a 0.5 grade point average the first semester. Testing of my true abilities and special attention from the dean of men at the University of Kentucky got me back on track. I was able to find a skill, journalism, and have a rewarding career.

I still lacked a solid sense of security, particularly in tight or uncertain situations. I was not a risk-taker. I wanted to know the outcome.

So my reaction to the cancer diagnosis in February 1997 was somewhat surprising to me.

The day after Dr. Rose called us with the diagnosis of multiple myeloma I kept the appointment in Elizabeth City.

I wanted the driving time to think and decide how I would deal with this, the greatest crisis of my life.

Based on my history, I truly expected to fall apart and become a basket case, as they say of someone who cannot deal with the shock of bad news.

Instead, I decided to fight the cancer with all that I had. I prayed and prayed. I returned home from the road trip with a goal of victory and was anxious to start chemotherapy.

I envisioned the pills sent out by Dr. Rose as little Pac-Men attacking the cancer in my body. I thought of the battle going on between the cancer cells and the chemo. I saw the chemo obliterating the bad cells. It was an image I would employ many times over the next ten months as we prepared for and then underwent the SCT.

I had a positive attitude throughout the rounds of chemo, aspirations, biopsies, infections, SCT and the recovery, including another infection that required hospitalization and then an IV drip at home for eight days.

ALICE: I was simply amazed at how positive Ambrose was. He never seemed worried or anxious. He, in fact, made me have a relaxed attitude. Otherwise, I would have been scared. He was so positive and relaxed that I felt OK, too!

It was his close relationship with God, our Father, that made all that possible, I'm sure.

AMBROSE: I kept asking myself, "Why am I so happy and so positive? This thing can kill me!"

Alice is right. The answer was my faith in God. I realized that my relationship with God was overcoming my natural tendency to panic and be a wimp.

I had developed in my early twenties a daily habit of at least thirty minutes of prayer and meditation. I was faithful to that regimen over the years. Everyone in the family knew that thirty minutes was God's time. I got out of bed before daylight to have a quiet time before the daily hustle and bustle of a young family trying to get ready for school and work.

Those daily sessions built a relationship with God and fortified me for the battle ahead. Alone I didn't have the strength to fight a major battle. God's strength overcame my weakness, as promised.

I had two occasions during the battle with cancer when I doubted.

Once was about 1:30 a.m. shortly after the diagnosis. I awoke and realized I wanted to get out of my body. I had learned to repeat the phrase "All is well. All is well with God." I said that to myself. The feeling left me almost immediately.

The second time was in the midst of the SCT after I had been given a lethal dose of chemo and two days of total body irradiation at UNC Hospitals. I was lying in my hospital bed when I questioned: "Do we really want to go through with this procedure?"

Again, I turned to "All is well. All is well with God." The feeling went away.

The people who surrounded us during the cancer treatment offered many prayers. People far and wide told us we were on their prayer lists. The support from family and friends buttressed our frequent prayers and my positive outlook.

I had never known my blood type. I was not surprised when the report came back at UNC Hospitals that it was B-positive.

I had a number of Bible verses and other quotations printed out to paste on the wall of my room during the transplant. I put one near my bed that said:

B +

...A cheerful heart has a continual feast.

Proverbs 15:15

I referred to it often along with one with the "all is well" quote and others that contained the following quotes:

Behold, I make all things new.

Rev. 21:5

— NOTHING CAN HURT —

God Calling, February 21

The way is plain.

You do not need to see far ahead. Just one step at a time with Me. The same light to guide you as the hosts of heaven know—the Son of Righteousness Himself.

Only self can cast a shadow on the way...

When you feel the absolute calm has been broken—away alone with Me until your heart sings and all is strong and calm.

— GO FORWARD —

God Calling, March 27

Rest in Me, quiet in My love, strong in My power. Think what it is to possess a power greater than any earthly force...

Go forward. You are only beginning the new Life together. Joy, joy, joy.

And then there was a thought in an *Upper Room* meditation I wish I had had during the SCT but didn't. I relied on it later as I worked to get well.

(Mark 4:40)

Jesus said to his disciples as waves pounded their small craft, "Why are you so afraid? Do you still have no faith?"

— THRILL OF PROTECTION —

God Calling, May 12

Turn out all thoughts of doubt and of trouble. Never tolerate them for one second. Bar the windows and doors of your souls against them as you would bar your home against a thief who would steal in to take your treasures.

What greater treasurers can you have than Peace and Rest and Joy? And these are all stolen from you by doubt and fear and despair. Face each day with love and laughter. Face the storm.

Joy, peace, love, My great gifts. Follow me to find all three. I want you to feel the thrill of protection and safety. Now. Any soul can feel this in a harbor, but real joy and victory come to those alone who sense these when they ride a storm.

Say "all is well." Say it not as a vain repetition. Use it as you use a healing balm for cut or wound, until the poison is drawn out; then, until the sore is healed; then until the thrill of fresh life floods your being.

All is well.

I went through the battle strengthened by those and other quotations and by the knowledge that God was with me whatever the outcome as Jesus was with the disciples during the turbulence in the boat.

Among the other books and readings that helped me was one book sent to me by two friends. It was so powerful that I bought copies to send to other cancer patients.

I think the philosophy contained in the book is a good model for anyone facing a serious illness or a major battle.

The book is titled *You Can't Afford the Luxury of A Negative Thought.* It is part of the Life 101 series and is authored by John-Roger and Peter McWilliams (Prelude Press, 1991).

John-Roger is an educator and McWilliams is a writer and poet.

It is a rich book that makes the following points:

"Thoughts have a power over our mind, our body and our emotions.

"Positive thoughts (joy, happiness, fulfillment, achievement, worthiness) have positive results (enthusiasm, calm, well-being, ease, energy, love). Negative thoughts (judgment, unworthiness, mistrust, resentment, fear) produce negative results (tension, anxiety, alienation, anger, fatigue)." (p. 13)

The authors say when a negative pattern is activated "we begin to look for everything wrong with a situation, person, place or thing. And we find it, too! There's always something wrong." (p. 24)

The negative thought pattern "puts a body through its paces. All the resources of the body are mobilized for immediate, physical, demanding action—fight or flee. All other bodily functions are put on hold—digestion, assimilation, blood cell production, body maintenance, circulation (except to certain vital skeletal muscles), healing and immunological responses…," the authors write.

They say that "for many negative thinking becomes a habit—a bad habit—which over time, degenerates into an addiction. It's a disease, like alcoholism, compulsive overeating or drug abuse." (p. 41)

The authors say we can question what we like, but "the accepted medical theory—that thoughts are a contributing factor of symptomatic illness and that improving one's thoughts can help improve one's health—is all we need to meet the premise of this book.

"The rest is, well, interesting, fun, provocative, stupid, enlightening—use your own adjectives to describe it. …it doesn't negate the fact that, in anyone's book—medical or metaphysical—if a life-threatening illness threatens, you can't afford the luxury of a negative thought." (p. 45)

The book talks about a cure for negative thinking, beginning with the knowledge that "you are the architect of your own cure."(p. 93)

"You can find ample evidence to prove your life is a miserable, depressing, terrible burden or you can find evidence to prove your life is an abundant, joyful, exciting adventure." (p. 129)

I thank God that I was sent the book. It helped me develop and put into words my positive attitude.

I continued to be surprised at my positive attitude. I thanked God for it and realized it came from Him. It wasn't me; it was His strength in me.

When I talk with other patients now, I stress how important a positive attitude was to my healing. And I point out that in some ways a positive attitude is selfish in that it is the most productive thing we can do to help in the healing process.

This is what my friend Jim Cheek told me as I began the battle. Jim had fought many recurrences of cancer. He had a very positive attitude. Despite the pain, Jim always had a smile on his face.

I visited Jim many times before he died. It was always a rich blessing to experience his positive attitude toward life. He helped me fight the battle by being a shining example of the love of Christ.

While Alice was going through her therapy we met others who had a positive attitude despite their serious medical problems.

One of these was Carlton Hicks, who had suffered four major strokes. He was like the Energizer Bunny—he kept on going.

After one stroke, Carlton had no feeling and no movement on his left side. The doctors said they hoped to get him out of the hospital in a couple of months and in time for Christmas.

Feeling returned and Carlton was discharged from the hospital in a matter of days.

He attributes his repeated recoveries from strokes to a positive attitude and trust in God.

Carlton, Alice, and I have commented often that we didn't see how anyone could successfully fight a major illness or injury without a strong faith in God.

We all know that our strongest position in fighting illness or injury is a positive attitude. And that strength comes from outside us.

My advice to those similarly situated is to

B +

NINE

God, my brain is all messed up. I don't know
what to pray for. You fix it anyway.

Prayer by Alice

AMBROSE: I was very peaceful during the SCT. I was not at peace when I became the caregiver for Alice. I also found I had little, if any, patience.

I think God uses situations to prune, or put another way, to improve His followers. Believe me, I was taught patience while caring for Alice. Some of it took. I had prayed for patience over the years.

"Be careful what you pray for; you probably will get it," pastors have warned me.

I actually worried about whether the demands on me were hurting my health. I did note that my heart rate went up during the periods of intense activity and frustration. My primary care doctor had me keep a log. While my blood pressure numbers were great, my heart rate climbed. It settled down when Alice finished intense therapy and we had time at home to rest and do what we wanted to do.

I do not for one moment discount the fact that this probably had to do, also, with a selfish streak. I tried hard to be the caring, loving husband and put my desires second. My psyche resisted and I think, on reflection, fighting this selfishness had a lot to do with my increased tension and heart rate.

Anyway, in August Alice began daily therapy at the WakeMed Outpatient Rehab facility. My journal shows I was tired all the time from the constant needs and demands. I had asked for some help in the morning to get Alice ready for rehab, but that help never came. It was all on me.

Alice said we could do it without help. That was easy for her to say.

After a month's experience of having the total responsibility, my diary shows it continued to wear me down. I was uptight and not very pleasant to be around. I asked God for more patience. I realized I was not cut out for this role.

ALICE: I'm surprised! I thought he was super.

AMBROSE: I don't know why I was so impatient—whether it was selfishness or tiredness from the cancer treatment. It was very upsetting to me and I cried a lot about the tiredness, stress and lack of patience. Alice was very understanding, becoming a reciprocal caregiver.

The lesson I learned from this and would suggest to other caregivers is: Take care of yourself, too!

We did win approval from the insurance carrier for a nurse's assistant to help care for Alice for twenty hours a week. This was mostly in the afternoon and one night a week. I pampered myself by continuing efforts to get a college degree at North Carolina Wesleyan College's Raleigh branch. I attended one class a week.

I should have insisted that more help be provided to drive Alice to rehab and to help meet her needs in the mornings.

The other side of this issue is what it does to the patient. Alice increasingly showed emotions over her condition and indications she was a burden to me.

She spontaneously became agitated about her condition and worried that she would not be a whole person again. Her inability to read because of double vision was a real concern.

During her hospital stay, we had an ophthalmologist examine her. He told me her eyes were good, but there had been nerve damage. He wanted to wait two months to give the eyes a chance to heal before prescribing a prism in her lens.

Alice agreed to the delay but was very frustrated.

We found there are a multitude of problems the patient and the primary caregiver face daily. The opportunity for frustration is great.

Anxiety was a big problem for Alice during her recovery in the hospital. She wanted to know exactly when visitors were going to arrive. If they weren't on time she would call the nurse's station. It was very difficult for me to deal with her anxiety because it appeared unfounded to me. To Alice it was very real.

We suggested that part of Alice's treatment plan include care for my psychological needs. This is often done through caregiver support groups, like the one Alice attended at UNC while I was undergoing treatment for cancer. These need to be conducted during the daytime as part of the weekly program. Suggestions for a caregivers' support group were met with "We leave that to this organization or that." It was the only failing we saw in the WakeMed rehab program.

Alice's routine involved daily sessions with physical, speech and occupational therapists. The recreational therapist oversaw aquatic sessions once or twice a week. Physical and recreational therapy continued after Alice was discharged from the daily program.

Amid all the demands and frustrations, we found some humor while Alice was an inpatient at WakeMed and while she was an outpatient at the rehab facility.

The nurses, therapists and nurses' assistants who cared for Alice became like members of the family, but Alice still had trouble getting her recovering brain to remember some names.

She referred to one nurse's assistant as "Vegetable" when she couldn't remember his name. He remains today one of her favorites. At other times she called therapists "the girls." Another therapist was called "Connie" although her name was Becky.

Alice also had trouble finding the right word in some situations. When an outing to a restaurant was planned, Alice objected because the location had not been picked by a therapist but by "one of the inmates" (patients).

That outing was a real confidence-builder for Alice. She awoke at 3 a.m. really upset and concerned the day of the trip. She was afraid of trying something new and had a list of excuses why the trip would not work.

In addition to the restaurant being picked by "one of the inmates," Alice reasoned:

- The "girls" (therapists) haven't seen it.
- The entrance might be uphill and hard for her to handle with a walker.

I talked with the therapist when we got to rehab that morning. She agreed they had not seen the restaurant but was confident the group could handle it. She pointed out to Alice that one of the reasons for the outing was to build confidence.

The trip went well for Alice. She had a good experience and was very proud of herself.

A week and a half later Alice began to walk indoors without the support of a cane or a walker. She still needed assistance outside because of vertigo which is not uncommon with brain injuries.

Alice's steps were deliberate because she didn't fully trust her left leg (it had been broken in the accident). She was getting more independent and became more helpful in doing household chores. She was beginning to regain her old role as mistress of the kitchen.

"Who rearranged *my* kitchen?" she asked one day in mid-September. I knew then she was making steady progress and wanted cooking utensils where she wanted them, not where I had put them.

Alice's mind was sharp, if not sharper than before. Her ability to analyze situations and her perceptions were fantastic. The occupational therapist had helped Alice work on her organization and planning skills—already an area she needed help with before the accident, but more severely needed afterward.

Dr. Mark Solomon, a clinical neuropsychologist at WakeMed Rehab, gave Alice a complete neuro workup in mid-October 1999 and found:

1. She had problems with short-term memory and some problems recalling long-term events.
2. Alice has trouble with speed of action, like starting to walk. She needed a few moments for the brain to get in gear.
3. Alice had trouble with complex problems, particularly when the method is changed in midstream.

But with those areas still needing attention, Dr. Solomon commented that "she is a miracle" considering where she had been and where she was at that moment. There was no other way to describe it.

Dr. Solomon said Alice would continue to improve her memory, speed of skills, and ability to handle complex issues. How far she would get, no one knows, he said.

"She is doing very, very well," he said.

Dr. Graham Snyder, who married Alice's niece Jane Hobson and was a new graduate of UNC Medical School, was a key caregiver from the beginning.

He told us during a later visit that he didn't think Alice would ever come out of the coma. Graham said the strong support from the family and conversations with Alice while she was comatose made a big difference.

During her recovery, I realized more than ever what a love Alice is. She is one of the sweetest people I have ever known. It is a pleasure being married to her and caring for her. I experienced great frustration because of the burden forced on me, but when I looked into her eyes I knew this was the role I really wanted.

Alice began to read more and rely less on the talking books that the state Services for the Blind provided after her dismissal from the hospital.

The double vision continued to bother her and did for another nine months until Dr. Robert Toler, an optometrist, found the right degree of prism for her glasses to make vertigo go away most of the time.

Alice also at this point was walking more without a cane and walker. She went from our garage about 30 feet to the street to talk with a neighbor, just holding onto my arm.

Unfortunately, this progress was not to last and by the next summer Alice had reverted to using the walker outside almost full-time. Her brother Fred figured out that she was afraid of falling on the pavement and hurting herself again. She was able to walk on the grassy lawn holding onto someone's arm.

Inside, Alice made steady progress in walking and by January 2000 was walking at a faster and more consistent pace. She said it felt like a switch had been thrown in her brain.

Outside she became agitated and sometimes had a full-blown panic attack when she stepped out of the car and faced walking on payment just holding onto someone's arms. Vertigo, again!

Dr. Patrick O'Brien, the primary rehab doctor, suggested we take a few weeks off from therapy around the Christmas holiday and come back to see him in January. We did and we appreciated the rest.

In January, Dr. O'Brien said Alice needed more physical therapy and he wanted to go "outside the box" of traditional medical rehab treatment and try neurofeedback.

Alice had eighty-five hours of neurofeedback with Drs. Dan Chartier and Lucy Potts in March, eleven months after the accident.

The treatment begins with an evaluation that includes an EEG (a map of the brain) and other diagnostics. The EEG showed severe brain injury from the left front to the right rear. The injury involved the shearing or severing of the axons, which tie the brain cells (neurons) to the nervous system.

The parts of the brain affected by the injury manage judgment, initiation, abstract thought, motor skills, sensory function, reading, writing, numbers and vision.

The treatment program is called the Life Quality Recovery Program (LQRP) and it seeks "to help persons with brain injuries reclaim a higher measure of quality in their lives."

Dr. Chartier explained that neurofeedback uses computer-assisted feedback technology to help the person improve brain function. The computer reads brain wave activity through a series of sensors placed on the patient's head.

"By teaching the brain to self-regulate abnormal brain wave patterns which have resulted from central nervous system injury, the brain can be altered into patterns which promote healthier behaviors," he said.

Chartier is a pioneer in the use of EEG neurofeedback. He began working with neurofeedback technology in 1990 and was elected president of the Society of Neuronal Regulation in 1999.

Dr. Chartier's office was located in a wooded setting on a major road west of Raleigh. Again, we were fortunate to have cutting-edge treatment near our home.

To reach the office we traversed a seventy-five-foot winding path through the woods, quite a challenge for a handicapped person. It took Alice seven and a half minutes to travel from the parking lot to the front door on the first visit.

We agreed that a test of the program's success would be the reduction in time needed to get from the parking lot to the door and whether she could do it holding onto a person's arm rather than a walker.

Alice began the actual neurofeedback March 28. She spent six hours a day, three days a week with Dr. Potts, who conducted the sessions most of the time. Alice had one intense week with Dr. Chartier three weeks after the initial visit while Dr. Potts was on vacation.

A touching moment came during the time of the neurofeedback treatments when Alice walked unassisted from the back pew to the front of North Raleigh United Methodist Church to take communion on Maundy Thursday. She broke into tears of joy as she returned to her pew. Pastor Billy Seate and members of the congregation who realized the significance of the event were teary-eyed, too. I was very proud of her.

One of the problems with Alice giving up the walker and going it on her own was a waviness in front of her eyes or dizziness she felt when she stood up. She said she often felt like she was drunk all the time. Alice said that led to a great deal of uncertainty. About four weeks into neurofeedback we began to see some major changes. The computer had been giving us data suggesting progress, but it took a while for her actions to reflect the change.

Dr. Potts said there were lots of "clinical moments," times when the data showed major progress.

"Come see this!" she would shout to Dr. Chartier.

On one of her days off from neurofeedback, Alice continued aquatic therapy. It was there one Friday that the therapist commented on how much better Alice was doing. Her walking in water, particularly backward, was very impressive.

Also, Alice walked down the pool's ramp without a cane or walker, just holding my hand. The next Sunday she walked into church holding my hand.

It showed how her initiative and confidence had improved during the neurofeedback sessions. And the icing on the cake was when she walked to and from LQRP, up and down the path, holding my hand. It took about three minutes one way.

It was a very satisfying feeling. But it didn't last. One day she froze when I tried to get her to walk outside holding my arm. She was locked up by fear that she would fall on the sidewalk or street. On the grass, she did fine. The street was another matter.

We had more work to do and another big mountain to conquer.

But neurofeedback had given Alice some of her greatest advances since the accident.

Dr. Solomon did another neuropsychological evaluation in August 2000. He found Alice "demonstrated quantifiable and remarkable cognitive improvement" since the October 1999 evaluation…. It should be noted that her psychomotor speed has appeared to have significantly increased as compared to her performance during the previous evaluation."

Not everything we tried worked for Alice. We weren't successful in our effort to solve the dizziness problem through a therapy that uses sounds, lights and motion.

Victories did continue to come, but slowly. Alice's initiative and confidence reached another milepost January 7, 2001. I was sick with a cold that day.

Alice drove herself to Sunday school. I sat next to the fireplace and praised the Lord for helping her over that big mountain.

My cheer had become: Go God, go!

I am convinced that the progress both of us made was due to our positive attitudes, the strong support of friends and loved ones and the fact that we kept God in the center of everything.

Being enveloped in the loving arms of caregivers does wonders for a patient struggling to be as normal as possible.

TEN

ALICE AND AMBROSE: The baskets hanging in the garage are a daily reminder of the love that came our way during our twin crises.

The baskets, elegant in their design, carried flowers, fruit, and goodies from dear friends. The baskets brought a strong message: We love and care for you.

The contents have been enjoyed, eaten or have wilted, but the memories of those random acts of kindness live on.

From time to time, we find a way to use one of those baskets to pass on God's love to someone else. It is the way sharing love works. The love we have felt uplifted us at the time we needed uplifting. Now it is our turn to pass that love on to others.

We were surrounded by abundant love as we fought the battle against cancer and struggled to heal from the head injury. The expressions of love seemed to come from everywhere. We were humbled by the number of people who took time to send us cards, flowers, food, and other gifts to show they cared.

A common theme was "You are in our thoughts and prayers. Hang in there!"

Some said more. All of the messages were uplifting. The two battles could not have been waged without the loving care of our friends, relatives and a God who met us at every turn.

There were those who took extra duties upon themselves. And there were those who said, "Let us know what we can do." All contributed to the care that sustained us during the hardest times of our lives. We were so richly blessed to have such support.

Dr. Seate, our pastor, was a constant source of strength, visiting us in the hospitals and at home. When we were homebound, Dr. Seate brought communion to our home between services on Sunday. His wife, Wanda, sent us the most wonderful and delicious sourdough bread she baked.

Frances Kunstling and Martha Gravely, two dear friends, established a list of people who asked to bring food. By sharing the responsibility of lining up meals, neither felt tied down by the duty. If one needed to be out of town, the other took over. It was a model for how to provide needed care on a daily basis without experiencing burnout.

Those two angels always will have a special place in our hearts. It is the kind of undying dedication and care that not only fills your stomach with great food, but also fills your heart with a warm glow of love.

One of the most appreciated acts of kindness was by a friend from Chapel Hill, Ann Henley, and her daughter, Caroline Davis. They came to our home, prepared dinner, served it and cleaned up. It was a delightful evening and gave us an "evening off" from kitchen duties.

We were on the prayer lists of churches in many states. There is no way to know how many people were praying for us, but we felt their prayers. We feel those prayers contributed to our healing.

There are scientific studies that support what we felt in our hearts.

Researchers at the Mid American Heart Institute, a program of St. Luke's Hospital in Kansas City, found heart patients who had someone praying over them, even without their knowledge, suffered 10 percent fewer complications than those who didn't. The study involved 990 patients admitted to the institute's coronary care unit during one year.

"It's potentially a natural explanation we don't understand yet. It's potentially a super- or other-than-natural mechanism," said William S. Harris, a heart researcher who was lead author of the study (AP, 10/25/99).*

Duke University researchers found a link between religion and good health. They said seniors with regular church or synagogue attendance are not only healthier but are less likely to die earlier than the irreligious.

The Duke study involved 4,000 people over 64 years old. It found the faithful were 28 percent less likely to die earlier compared to those who didn't attend religious services or didn't attend regularly.

"These studies do not show that if they are going to church for health reasons, their health will improve. But if people go to church for religious reasons, they have better health and survive longer," said Dr. Harold Koenig, the study's lead author (AP, 7/22/99).*

The *News & Observer* of Raleigh reported in July 1999 that physicians and nurses are no longer limited to cold and sterile offices. Churches are sponsoring volunteer teams of personal trainers and health care professionals.

"More and more, parish nurses and congregational health ministries are seizing upon the growing connection between faith and healing by assuming visible roles in faith communities that help address the gaps that traditional health care models are missing," the *News & Observer* reported.

In addition, the paper reported that hospitals such as WakeMed in Raleigh and UNC Hospitals in Chapel Hill are funding parish nursing programs in faith communities.

"I think that faith-based institutions have understood for a long time that you can't separate faith and health," said Nancy Rago-Durbin, coordinator of parish nursing special projects for the International Parish Nurse Resource Center in Parkridge, Ill.

"Hospitals may not be addressing anything more than their [the patients'] physical health. A church has such a wonderful opportunity to say, 'We care about all of you.' And when you watch and read and look at literature, people are starting to hear and believe in the power of prayer and healing" (Joyce Clark Hicks, "Prayer & Care," E1, *The News & Observer*, July 1, 1999).

We certainly experienced many saying, "We care about all of you."

There was a genuine concern for the total person by most of the nurses when Alice and I were hospitalized. The coordinators in the bone marrow transplant program and the rehab facilities were particularly concerned that the patient and the family received loving care.

The hospitals' staffs were wonderful to Alice and me. They made us feel like family. Friendships developed during hospital stays continue years later.

Those outside the health care community were sensitive not to "bother us." That is essential in providing care, particularly when a person is hospitalized. Visits can be uplifting to the patient, but they can also be exhausting.

We learned there is an art to having a meaningful and productive hospital visit. The visit should be no longer than 10 minutes unless the patient suggests you stay longer.

Many called before visiting to see if we were up to having company in the hospital.

"I would enjoy a short visit" was my standard reply.

Not all honored my request. One friend came and stayed ninety minutes. I was tired and needed a nap, but I didn't want to be rude. He eventually ran out of steam and left.

A patient should not be put in the position of feeling he or she must entertain a visitor. The patient is in the hospital to get well, not hold an open house. Of course, nurses can be asked to graciously run interference for the patient. They are very tactful in finding something that needs to be done at that very moment.

Generally, we found people respected the patient's time and energy level. Most expressed their love by a card or gift. One of the editors at the AP Raleigh office, Martha Waggoner, brought a very special gift one afternoon: A milk shake from the Char-Grill restaurant. It was a refreshing relief from the boredom of hospital food.

We saved the cards and letters we received. Looking back at those brings a warm reminder of how much people cared.

We reproduce here a sampling to give the flavor of the circle of care we experienced.

"Keep your chin up, buddy, and never feel alone. We are plugging for you—and for your family." (A newspaper colleague in western North Carolina)

"Sorry to hear about your accident. Get back to school quick. We have lots to talk about." (A student Alice counseled)

"Words cannot express my sorrow over this tragic accident. As you already know, Alice is a wonderful, wonderful, wonderful counselor and human being. I would be honored to help you and your family in any way possible." (A school principal)

"I know there's nothing I can say and do to make it better. But I hope you take comfort in the love and prayers of all your many friends. Take care of yourself and know that we're out there rooting for you."(An AP colleague in the West)

"The gang worldwide is pulling for you." (A New York coworker)

Humor always was welcome.

"Is it true the hospital is cutting costs by using coin-operated bedpans?" (A colleague in Tennessee)

One colleague sent tapes from old radio comedy shows.

"We have you at the top of the list of nightly prayers, so be assured you are being mentioned in dispatches on the Heavenly Internet." (A colleague in the Northeast)

The cards were hopeful and upbeat.

"We media folks don't talk much about God, faith, spirituality and prayer. I guess we're somehow afraid that those areas are without tangible documentation. And, how do you attribute a physical triumph over scientific nadir? Maybe we posture in those ways in order to protect our vulnerability to things unexplained and unexplainable. At any rate, my friend, I know that God does perform miracles and that prayer works." (A colleague in North Carolina)

"You give so much of yourself to others in bringing the love of Christ to everyone you meet. May God be with you in your time of need and give you the strength to go through with your treatments. Our prayers are with you." (Sheets Day Care Center where I meditate weekly with shut-ins).

During my illness, my AP chief of bureau colleagues met in New York. Some arranged a special prayer service for me. The hospitality room was turned into a chapel. They sent me a video of the occasion.

A couple in our Raleigh church was in the congregation of a New England church when a woman asked everyone to pray for a friend of hers in Raleigh, Alice Dudley. Our church members were pleasantly surprised to see the army of God working for a friend in another state.

Expressions of love like this sampling make a big impact in the life of someone struggling to regain health. They uplift the patient and the patient's family.

ELEVEN

Cast all your anxieties on Him, for He cares about you.

1 Peter 5:7

AMBROSE: One Sunday morning during the fifteen-month respite between my returning to work and Alice's accident, we were driving through the western Piedmont listening to a radio minister from Calvary Baptist Church in New York City preach on 1 Peter 5:7. He listed four factors in turning your cares over to God.

We soon realized the points in his sermon paralleled our experience when I was being treated for cancer and undergoing the SCT. We followed the same list in dealing with Alice's injury and recovery. It became a way of life for us.

The minister talked about *thankfulness, helpfulness, decisiveness,* and *trustfulness.*

It wasn't the order in which I would have put the list, but his message had a familiar ring. The idea of God's peace had been just a concept to me, but I came to know personally what Paul called the peace that passes understanding.

A bone marrow or stem cell transplant is a serious medical procedure. It allows the doctors to give the body enough chemotherapy and, in my case, total body irradiation to hopefully destroy the cancer.

The bone marrow is killed, and the white blood cell count drops to 100 or below as compared to the normal 4,000 to 10,500. The immune system is destroyed.

Amidst this uncomfortable and, frankly, somewhat frightening procedure, I experienced total peace. While I sat in the hospital room, I asked, "Why am I so peaceful ... so happy? This could kill me."

"Because I am here," was His answer. God has been with us every step of the way from the night my oncologist told us I had multiple myeloma through seven rounds of chemotherapy, four days of total body irradiation and the ongoing recovery.

A positive attitude that allows the body to do the healing work God intended is one of the major contributions a patient can make to the treatment process.

The radio preacher's sermon brought to mind some of our faith experience in fighting this aggressive disease.

THANKFULNESS: We were not thankful for the disease, but we were very thankful that we didn't have to go through the battle alone. God was there, giving His peace. Every morning I repeated that familiar verse: "This is the day the Lord has made; let us rejoice and be glad in it."

There were three writings that served especially as a source of strength. Two were from the daily mediation book *God Calling*, written by two unidentified women in England who heard the voice of Christ, and the other was Margaret Fishback Powers' wonderful "Footprints," which I posted on my wall in the hospital room.

Even with those inspirational works, I always found it strange that I wasn't in a panic during the SCT since most of my life involved uncertainty after uncertainty and a scared, choking sensation in tight situations. It truly was the peace that passes all understanding.

HELPFULNESS: What did we learn from this experience about ourselves? How did we grow? What can we use from this experience to help others?

God has given us a number of opportunities to share with others who are either facing a bone marrow transplant, a closed head injury or a struggle with cancer. Some are doing well; others didn't make it. But we knew it was no accident that we found ourselves with the opportunity to share.

Talking with someone who has faced death has a way of helping a patient deal with the situation. I was eager to be helpful to others because I knew what it meant to receive the help of someone else. Jim Cheek's beautiful, positive attitude was my shining example.

"You do what you've got to do and just trust God," Jim would tell me. Then he would talk about the goodness of life. It was an uplifting moment. I knew I had been given a special gift from Jim. I wanted to share that gift with others.

DECISIVENESS: I made a decision to cast my cares upon the Lord. When Dr. Rose was getting ready to do the first bone marrow aspiration for a biopsy, I thought of Christ on the cross. I said: "If you can handle that, I can handle this." I thought many times of the scene of Christ dying for me and the Resurrection that followed.

I decided to rely on His power, recognizing that we were not equipped to deal alone with life's most trying times. That is not the time to try to be a superhero. It is time to assess where you are in life, what you want out of life, what is really important and who is really important. For me, the most important thing in my life is my relationship with God. Out of that all other relationships grow.

If I really meant that I trusted God, then I needed to trust Him! I did and it made the difference. It is a crucial step in allowing the body to do what it wants to do and what God intended for it to do: participate in the healing process.

Trusting God doesn't mean the situation necessarily will turn out the way you would like for it to. I knew from the start that I could die during my treatment. We knew Alice could die as a result of her head injury.

My analysis of my situation was this: If I die healthy, I will be with God. If I die sick, I will be with God. So either way I am going to end up in the same place. I don't need to spend my energy worrying about that. I need to do my part to get well.

I took Jim's advice, trusted God and kept on keeping on.

TRUSTFULNESS: I trusted God to be who He said He was. I was determined not to try to dictate to God. I trusted Him with the future regardless of how the battle with cancer was going to end. Once I released my concerns to Him, I worked hard not to try to reclaim them. When fears would enter in, I would repeat the words from a meditation: "All is well. All is well" with God by my side.

It is very hard not to try to reclaim your concerns after turning them over to God. It is only human to want to run things. It becomes easier to trust your doctor, your body and God when you realize it is in your best interest to do that. Trying to be a superhero could be the one thing that leads to serious trouble.

ALICE: Ambrose was so relaxed and at such peace that one would have thought he was going on a Sunday school picnic instead of having a transplant. I would have been anxious and nervous, but he was so much at peace that I felt relaxed and confident.

There was only one night when I left the hospital feeling a little uneasy about Ambrose's condition. I called when I arrived at my brother's house, talked with Ambrose and was reassured that he was feeling better and ready for "bed."

Ambrose was an inspiration not only to me, but also to everyone who talked to one of us. I really think his faith and his good spirit had an enormous effect on his recovery. His rapid progress was certainly not the norm; people were amazed at how well he did and at how quickly he progressed.

AMBROSE: I am in a remission. Alice is continuing to heal slowly. We don't know how long my remission will last or how much healing Alice will experience. We do know that God is with us, sharing His love and His peace.

After the transplant, one of our friends called to express concern. She spoke in a whisper as she asked about my condition.

"He's doing very well," Alice said. "Things are looking good."

Alice got off the phone and asked, "Is there something wrong with us? Everyone else is so down and we are so happy!"

TWELVE

AMBROSE: It seems that all of our life together Alice and I have met life hand in hand as a couple. I sensed that she would be a partner and would help me be better than I was. That is one of the primary reasons I married her. This was in contrast to other relationships I had had.

When Alice and I met in 1963, I was ending a courtship with a woman from California. There was a major conflict between her Roman Catholic beliefs and mine as a United Methodist. I wanted children to be free to choose their religion. She wanted to tie them to the Catholic Church. Our friendship did not withstand that storm, which became very intense at times.

I sought a person with similar religious beliefs. At the time, I didn't fully realize how important that was in my life. I had not come to understand that the most important relationship in my life was my relationship with God.

Alice and I met at Dilworth UMC, where she was working with Pastor Robinson. A deep friendship quickly developed, and I decided to tell my friend from California it just wasn't going to work.

"You will thank God a million times for this," Pastor Robinson said to me sitting in his parlor when I told him the other relationship had ended and I wanted to date Alice. I had talked with him a number of times about the conflict over allowing children to be free to choose their religious affiliation.

His words were prophetic. I have thanked God many, many times for Alice as we have gone step-by-step, hand in hand through forty-two years of marriage that included many moves, rearing two fine sons, enjoying five granddaughters and two daughters in law and dealing with our dual crises.

Sadly, Pastor Robinson was fighting his own battle with cancer at the time we spoke. He later died. His failing strength did allow him to preach one last great sermon to the Dilworth congregation. He passed the collection plate twice during the service. Some said he passed the plate twice because he was getting forgetful as the disease took over his body. I never believed that for a moment. He knew what he was doing. He always talked about passing the plate twice. It was his last chance and he did it.

The sense of humor he showed during those dark hours was always an inspiration to me. I thought of it while I was in the midst of the transplant. It made me laugh.

The relationship Alice and I have has grown from those first dates when we both knew—but didn't say to each other—that we had found our mate for life. During premarriage counseling, Dr. Tuttle set the tone for our being able to handle the many trials and crises that touched our marriage.

He was right that we were creating something brand new and that the new family, partnership, team, twosome, or whatever you wanted to call it was ours and God's.

If we kept God in the relationship as a full participating partner, the marriage would make it through the trials.

We grew closer and stronger in our faith as we met each challenge.

A successful marriage takes a lot of work by both parties. And it takes a lot of forgiveness and swallowing pride. We grew together.

Alice had lots of work to do in polishing me and making me a better person and partner. I don't think I really started growing out of my selfish tendencies until I cared for her following the traffic accident. I know I learned a great deal of patience in those months. God has a wonderful way of using situations to refine a person.

Alice was always a loving, forgiving, outgoing person everyone loved immediately. Her smile and pleasant demeanor made her a wonderful director of Christian education and later a guidance counselor. She is the best wife.

Of course, our marriage went through the normal trials and strains. We struggled to make it work and early on made a rule that we would never go to sleep at night angry with each other and we would always say "I love you" before parting in the morning.

Knowing that we had said "I love you" as the last thing the morning of Alice's accident gave me great comfort as we drove to Durham to see her in the hospital.

Our marriage met its first major trial when we decided it was time to have children and had trouble conceiving. We considered the alternatives, prayed, underwent examination after examination, and eventually found that I was the problem.

It was three years between the time we decided to have a family and the day Alice announced that we were pregnant.

Our struggle to start a family and going through childbirth education classes and the delivery together provided a great bonding experience. We learned to work as a team.

When I was diagnosed with multiple myeloma, it was natural that it was "our" disease and it would be "our" fight. There was no other way to handle it.

The first few months involved dealing with the shock of the diagnosis, planning the course of treatment and dealing with the mechanics of one partner being sidelined by a major illness.

Alice was my coach, my advocate and my companion during the SCT. Her pleasant smile and happy approach, even in the midst of this trial, uplifted me every time she came into the room. When the days were the darkest and we didn't know whether I would engraft or not, her mere presence gave me hope.

We both looked for the humor in the situation. In the days when I felt the worst and hurt the most, Alice kept my spirits up by telling me what was going on outside my room.

One day she overheard a conversation between the husband of the patient next door and the nurse who was trying to deliver a tray of food.

"My wife don't want no food. My wife don't want to smell no food. My wife don't even want to know no food exists," Alice reported the husband saying to the nurse.

I knew the feeling. I didn't want any food and particularly I "didn't want no coffee" in those maroon plastic cups. The only thing that made me sick during the whole SCT was cold, decaf coffee in a plastic cup. Today, I still get a sick feeling in my stomach when I see such a cup.

The burden was all on Alice to take care of the house, pay the bills and manage things while I was in the hospital. She had to adapt to my system since there wasn't time to develop her own.

She had her hands full when it became clear that I was going to be released much sooner than originally anticipated. The house had to be cleaned, all plants removed and preparations made for a husband who had an immune system that was shaky at best.

We left UNC Hospitals on October 3 and started my second life hand in hand.

It was a year and a half later that the roles would be reversed.

As Alice lay in Duke Hospital in a coma, our friend Dee Bostick said to me in her best counselor voice: "Well, Ambrose it is your turn now (to be the caregiver)."

Alice and I had discussed many times what we would do if one of us were ill and could not speak. When her Aunt Sadie was hospitalized following a stroke, Alice tried to speak for her and it meant a great deal to her relatives.

"You know what I would want to say," Alice told me driving home from visiting her Aunt Sadie in the hospital in Winston-Salem. "I would want to say 'I love you,' and I would want to know how you are doing and the children."

We practiced a little handholding exercise where she squeezed my hand and I squeezed hers to the words:

I (squeeze) love (squeeze) you (squeeze, squeeze).

We did it over and over again on the way home and many times thereafter.

I had a ritual when I visited the comatose Alice in the hospital in Durham and in Raleigh. The first thing I did when I arrived was to take her hand and squeeze, saying "I (squeeze) love (squeeze) you (squeeze, squeeze). You (squeeze) love (squeeze) me (squeeze, squeeze)" over and over again.

Next, if I could keep the medical people and visitors out of the room long enough, we would have a time of meditation. I would read from the *Upper Room*, a daily devotional book used by many United Methodists, from the book titled *God Calling*, the Bible and other material.

I would repeat the 23rd Psalm, one of Alice's favorites, and other verses from the Bible followed by a prayer. Then we would "talk." I would tell her what was going on in our world.

Alice remembered nothing from those "talks."

During the day and at night, other members of the family and some friends would gather around Alice's bed and "talk" with her. She had verbal stimulation from 10 a.m. to 8 p.m. or longer, if we were permitted to stay.

We also encouraged her to squeeze our hand if she heard us or to move a part of her body. We thought there was some movement on occasion, but that may have been wishful thinking.

Even if there wasn't movement, we wanted to try every way to stimulate her.

Medical people have told us that those conversations with Alice while she was in a coma made a big difference in her recovery. The theory is that although she didn't remember any of it, she subconsciously knew she was not alone and was loved very much.

THIRTEEN

ALICE: The skills we developed while working together on life's difficulties help us face the future with great optimism. Life goes on. We have a lot of living we want to do.

We are both physically challenged—I in a more ambulatory way than Ambrose, whose activities are limited by profound fatigue. I have vertigo when standing and use a walker to maintain balance. We must live with those challenges.

But we plan to live as full a life as possible, allowing for our difficulties and deficiencies. We attend the symphony, go out to dinner with friends and travel.

During our recoveries, we have taken trips to Ambrose's home state, Kentucky, and to Ireland and England, which we had planned to visit the summer of my accident. We took three cruises to the Caribbean and a trip to the Canadian Rockies and Alaska.

We don't want to feel sorry for ourselves and just sit around the house moaning and groaning about how our disabilities won't allow for fun. We don't think it is healthy to concentrate on the things a person can't do. We want to find new and creative ways to do things. Sometimes it is hard work.

When we travel, for instance, it takes major planning. Because of fatigue Ambrose cannot drive long distances like he used to do in his work. I drive some now, but very little on the interstate highways.

We get around our "driving problems" by taking short trips and getting others to do the driving.

If we drive, we plan to start early and stop early. If we fly, we call the airline and make arrangements for a wheelchair for me. We find that it is easier to have a wheelchair at our disposal. I don't normally use a wheelchair, but using one at airports means things move along more quickly and smoothly since we sometimes have a long trek to the gate.

We want to look at the glass as half full instead of half empty. As someone said once: "You do what you can with what you've got."

That philosophy of dealing with our deficiencies is rooted in our religious faith and the training I had as a guidance counselor. It leaves us with a positive attitude in facing difficulties.

I studied a number of theorists in graduate school and in various workshops. Some of that training was in Reality Therapy under Dr. William Glasser and Perry Goode.

In another workshop about the Myers-Briggs personality inventory, I was told that each person has preferences. My training taught that a person can make choices about how to lead his or her life, regardless of the person's background or current situation.

Reality Therapy used the model of a car. The front wheels represented thinking and doing. The rear wheels represented feelings and emotions.

The question is: What drives you? Do you confront problems with your emotions and feelings or do you think through the situation and then plan how to deal with it?

We have learned that front-wheel-drive cars do better in snow and mud than vehicles propelled by rear wheel drive.

Dr. Glasser taught us that a person must face the realities of his or her situation. Do what you can do.

Ambrose and I also are always thankful for what we have and what we have received. We feel there have been many miracles in both of our recoveries. Others have confirmed this.

We thank a loving God every morning for life itself and how He has blessed us in the midst of our difficulties.

We want to look ahead and not back. We have mountains to climb. Some we will not be able to climb. We will go as far as we can and not dwell on those hills we can't conquer.

Ambrose, who made a 0.5 grade point average his first college semester, climbed one big hill in getting a BS degree. He resumed his education late in life and graduated with honors from North Carolina Wesleyan in 2000.

I feel compelled to say a little about those mountains we can't climb lest the reader think everything is peaches and cream.

Sometimes I do get a little discouraged. From what we have written, readers may think we are happy all the time. We are not Pollyannas, but real people with real problems.

Most of the time, we look on the bright side of life. Sometimes, however, there are discouraging times.

When I am out in a crowded place, I see people walking around and I ask myself "Why can't I walk like that?" It seems so natural for others, but here I am with my walker. After a few moments of discouragement, I realize how very fortunate I am.

I am alive, and I have my loving husband, wonderful family and caring friends. I really am most blessed.

Ambrose, too, has his moments of discouragement. He sees our neighbors, doing "normal" thinks like going on long walks, traveling to the beach regularly, and so on. Fatigue limits his level of activity. It is hard for us to do things spontaneously.

We used to take a two-mile walk several times a week. Now, we can't. We miss that time together. Our hearts say "yes," but our bodies say, "not now."

We must adjust to the realities of our lives. We get discouraged, but we pull out of it by looking at what we have rather than what we don't have.

Dr. Rose, Ambrose's oncologist, gave us a lift six years after his diagnosis. During one of our thrice-annual checkups, Dr. Rose told Ambrose his blood work, lungs, and everything else looked good.

"Where do we go from here?" Ambrose asked.

"I don't know; I haven't had anyone live this long without the disease coming back," Dr. Rose said.

We look on life as a gift. I am writing this as we drive to my sister's house on the coast. My once-legible handwriting has turned to chicken scratch, and I tire easily. Plus Ambrose has to try to read my scratching when he types on the computer.

But that is the life we must live. Nobody ever told us life was fair. To worry about that, we feel, is to cry over spilled milk, as our mothers would say. We want to look forward.

We have always said we don't know what the future holds, but we know Who holds the future.

As long as we have on this earth, we will face the future hand in hand with each other and with God, our loving caregiver.

BIBLIOGRAPHY

BOOKS

Holy Bible, Revised Standard Version, New York: Thomas Nelson & Sons, 1952.

John-Roger and Peter McWilliams, *You Can't Afford the Luxury of a Negative Thought*. Los Angeles: Prelude Press, 1991.

Robinson, Harold M., *Happy … If with My Latest Breath: Sermons of a Man Facing Death*. N.p.: Privately printed by the author's family, n.d.

Russell, A. J., ed., *God Calling & God at Eventide*, New York: Dodd, Mead, & Company, 1950; reprint 1978.

ARTICLES

Abbott, John S. "Caregiver's Handbook," American Share Foundation, 1995.

"Caring for the Caregiver," *Wellness Letter*, University of California, Berkeley, December 2000, p. 4.

Coleman, Brenda, "Power of Prayer," The Associated Press, October 25, 1999.

"Helping the Patient by Helping the Caregiver," *Johns Hopkins Medical Letter*, July 2000, p. 3.

Hicks, Joyce, "Prayer and Care," *The News & Observer*, July 1, 1999, p. 1, sec. E.

Robertson, Gary, "Religion-Health," The Associated Press, July 22, 1999.

"Seek and Accept Help," *OncoLink BMT Newsletter*, Issue 37, February 1997.

"Set Up a Support System for You," *OncoLink BMT Newsletter*, Issue 37, February 1997.

"Surviving the Transplant Experience—The Caregiver's Perspective, Part II," *OncoLink BMT Newsletter*, Issue 37, February 1997.

"What Is Myeloma?" International Myeloma Foundation, Myeloma.org, 1996.

ABOUT THE AUTHORS

Alice and Ambrose Dudley live in Raleigh, North Carolina, with their dog Grady. They have five lovely granddaughters: Emily, Hannah, Grace, Abigail and Avery.